浙江省普通高校"十三五"新形态教材

ENGLISH
OF LIBERAL ARTS FOR STUDENTS
OF HEALTH SCIENCE

医疗通识英语

主 编 崔 红 洪 洋

副主编 陈 一 严 挺 龙天娇

ZHEJIANG UNIVERSITY PRESS
浙江大学出版社

Preface
前　言

　　《医疗通识英语》是浙江省普通高校"十三五"新形态教材，是根据国家教育事业发展"十三五"规划、教育部颁布的《大学英语课程要求》《高等职业教育英语课程教学要求》编写的顺应"互联网+"教育信息化时代背景的创新实用立体化特色教材。教材内容涵盖医疗卫生、健康服务等领域相关的通识英语知识技能、跨文化交际和自主学习策略等。

　　本教材主要针对高等教育阶段医学类、卫生类院校的实际教学需求而编写，同时满足医疗、健康服务领域广大从业人员继续学习的需求，以助其完成多元知识储备与技能提升，创造更优的人才经济附加值。

　　《医疗通识英语》全面融入社会主义核心价值观，积极传播中国传统健康文化，唯物辩证地汲取西方先进文化，通过一版和二版的实践探索，进一步明确了新时期教材的全新内涵，有机融合"新形态"元素和"课程思政"元素，为最终实现以社会主义核心价值观引领的职业素养与英语技能兼备的人才培养目标而努力。

　　《医疗通识英语》充分对接"职教二十条"的要求，深入思考以学习者为中心的教法与学法的统一，采用多媒融合的数字资源开发、学生泛在学习空间建设等手段，重点突破不同学习者的个性化学习需求的难题，通过信息技术与英语语言教学的深度融合，实现学习者与教材资源的共同"成长"，使教材的应用更有利于激发学习者的自主学习兴趣，从而有效促进课堂改革创新和课程活力提升。教材表现形式丰富，教材与教学、线上与线下紧密结合，充分呈现"新形态"特点。

　　一是基于全生命周期理念的医疗健康通识英语主题设计。

　　面向全生命周期的医疗健康通识英语知识与技能，注重社会主义核心价值观引领，以全人关怀、医护职业素养、跨文化交际能力和学习策略为主要内容编写实用特色教材，通过六个章节，强化六大核心内容：（1）预防保健常识，如疫情防控与急救知识；（2）思想意识形态，如中国医养文化的传承与传播；（3）全球医护视野，涉及全球化的医护行业与教育；（4）全人生命关爱，如全生命周期与医护人文；（5）未来健康服务，如关注全球老龄化趋势与幼儿发展；（6）美好生活理念，如生活美容艺术等。本教材既有传承，又有发扬，并以语言工具为探索新世界的手段，将有助于潜移默化地培养学生对知识鉴赏的品位、文化思辨的意识、技能创新的精神。

二是基于多媒融合理念的新形态数字资源设计。

如何在外语信息化教学语境中更好地实现"教"的各要素与"学"的各维度之间协同发展，是本教材开发、编写过程中致力破解的难题。在呈现形式方面，本新形态教材大胆突破，对数字资源的开发与利用进行创新，使"新形态"的特点体现在具体问题的解决上，即读者在与资源的共同"成长"中，实现对于多媒融合知识的按需索取（On-Demand Inquiry，ODI）。在教材内容方面，本新形态教材充分结合课程思政融入的需求，以英语工具培养"带进来"与"走出去"的自信；跨平台的新形态教材在淡化"书本"媒介属性的同时，不断强化外语知识的实践用途，最佳匹配"动态"的教学需求。如何实现资源"按需分配（On-Demand Assignment，ODA）"一直是传统教材及第一代电子教材"功能论"的讨论焦点。借由教材数字资源在方式与内涵上的双重升级，该问题迎刃而解，并在教材开发的过程中，经过了课程改革与课堂教学实践案例的验证。

结合全新自主研发的 TRAMS 诠识外语资源库及在线课程，本教材实现了富媒体数字资源跨平台整合与全时段调用。读者可利用书中丰富的二维码，实时接入这座不断更新的数字化知识宝库，获取本书配套的视频、音频、字幕、文本、演示、动画、案例、图谱、题库、答案等资源，与全球用户全程分享快乐学习体验。

通过课前扫码预热，学习者重新认识国医精粹，激发用英语"走出去"的文化自信；在课中扫码深入学习，实现国际先进医疗通识"带进来"的学习目的；最后，在课外进入 TRAMS 外语微信公众号阅读精选原版英文材料，有效延伸课堂内容，让学习者以"已知"探索"未知"，以丰富的全数字外文语料，激发"新体验"，习得"新知识"。

综上所述，《医疗通识英语》在使用设计上贯穿"课前—课中—课后"的完整学习过程，实现了 ODA 到 ODI 的范式转变，较传统方式更加灵活；教材内容的自定义性更强，资源与教材的适切性更好，不但完全适用于传统方式英语课堂的教学创新，也符合大数据时代"泛在学习"的趋势与要求，具备较强的实用性、适用性与创新性。建议读者在使用中根据具体需求，结合自身专业背景、职业取向、语言基础、教学策略及课时计划特点，进行个性化的章节内容选取，以实现最佳教学效果。

由于编者水平有限，编写过程中疏漏与错误在所难免，恳请读者与同行不吝指正。

编 者

2020 年 3 月

CONTENTS
目　录

Chapter 1

Health Guardian

健康卫士

Unit 1 Epidemic Hazards: Prevention Is Better Than Cure

防优于治

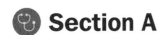 ## Section A

Video 1-1

Warm-up Activity【疫问医答　权威发布】

In this video(Video 1-1) the World Health Organization (WHO) explains the basic knowledge of coronavirus (冠状病毒). Discuss with group members the questions and answers involved, and then conclude what you understand based upon the discussion. Present your ideas with no more than 20 words in English.

Here is an example:

Coronaviruses can be transmitted between animals and humans, and to protect ourselves we should wash our hands properly. (18 words)

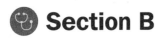 ## Section B

Ⅰ Graphic Advice: Whats & Hows【抗击疫情　远离传染】

Novel Coronavirus (2019-nCoV) Advice for the Public

A novel (新型的) coronavirus (CoV) is a new strain (种类) of coronavirus that has not been previously identified (识别) in humans. 2019-nCoV is from the same family of viruses as Severe (重症的) Acute (急性) Respiratory (呼吸系统的) Syndrome (综合征) (SARS-CoV)，but it is not the same virus. The new, or "novel" coronavirus, now called 2019-nCoV, had not previously detected before the outbreak (暴发) was reported in Wuhan, China in December 2019.

As with other respiratory illnesses, infection (感染) with 2019-nCoV can cause mild (轻度的) symptoms including a runny nose, sore throat (咽喉炎), cough, and fever. It can be more severe for some persons and can lead to pneumonia (肺炎) or breathing difficulties. More rarely, the disease can be fatal (致命的). Older people, and people with pre-existing medical conditions (such as asthma(哮喘), diabetes, heart disease) appear to be more vulnerable (虚弱的) to becoming severely ill with the virus.

People of all ages can be infected by the new coronavirus. Older people, and people with pre-existing medical conditions appear to be more vulnerable to becoming severely ill with the virus. According to recent reports, it may possible that people infected with 2019-nCoV may be infectious before showing significant (明显的) symptoms. However, based on currently available data, the people who have symptoms are causing the majority of virus spread. Be aware that the incubation (潜伏期) period (the time between infection and the onset（发病）of clinical symptoms of disease) of 2019-nCoV could be up to 14 days.

WHO advises people of all ages to take steps to protect themselves from the virus. WHO's standard recommendations (建议) for the general public to reduce exposure to and transmission (传播) of a range of illnesses are as follows, which include hand and respiratory hygiene (卫生), and safe food practices.

（1）Protect yourself and others from getting sick.

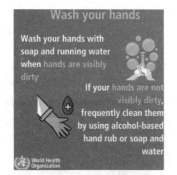 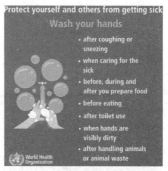

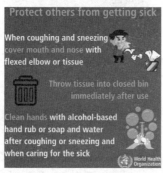 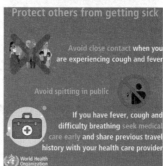

（2）Practise food safety.

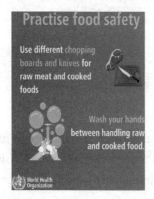 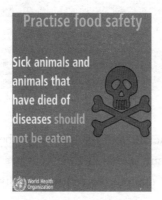 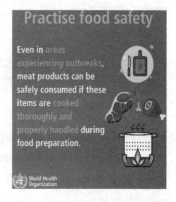

(*Source*: WHO, January 2020)

Ⅱ Notes【说文解字　名词注释】

1. Vocabulary Table

🎧 Vocabulary 1-1

Words & Expressions	Part of Speech	Meaning in Text
epidemic	*adj.*	流行病的
coronavirus	*n.*	冠状病毒
novel	*adj.*	新型的；新颖的
strain	*n.*	品种；（疾病的）类型；株
identify	*vt.*	辨识；识别
severe	*adj.*	严重的；重症的
acute	*adj.*	急性的
respiratory	*adj.*	呼吸的；呼吸系统的
syndrome	*n.*	综合病征；综合症状；症候群
SARS	*n.*	非典型性肺炎
outbreak	*n.*	爆发
infection	*n.*	感染
mild	*adj.*	轻度的
sore throat	*phr.*	咽喉炎；喉咙痛
pneumonia	*n.*	肺炎
fatal	*adj.*	致命的
diabetes	*n.*	糖尿病
vulnerable	*adj.*	虚弱的；易感的
asthma	*n.*	哮喘
significant	*adj.*	明显的；显著的
incubation	*n.*	潜伏期；孵化
onset	*n.*	发病；发生
recommendation	*n.*	推荐；建议
transmission	*n.*	传播
hygiene	*n.*	卫生

2. Useful Knowledge

(1) The animal source of the 2019-nCoV has not yet been identified. This does not mean you can catch 2019-nCoV from any animal or from your pet. To protect yourself, when visiting live animal markets, avoid direct unprotected contact with live animals and surfaces in contact with animals.

The consumption of raw or undercooked animal products should be avoided. Raw meat, milk or animal organs should be handled with care, to avoid cross-contamination with uncooked foods, as per good food safety practices.

At present there is no evidence that companion animals or pets such as cats and dogs have been infected or have spread 2019-nCoV.

(2) People with 2019-nCoV infection, the flu, or a cold typically develop respiratory symptoms such as fever, cough and runny nose. Even though many symptoms are alike, they are caused by different viruses. Because of their similarities, it can be difficult to identify the disease based on symptoms alone. That's why laboratory tests are required to confirm if someone has 2019-nCoV. Do note that antibiotics do not work against viruses—they only work on bacterial infections. The novel coronavirus is a virus and, therefore, antibiotics should not be used as a means of prevention or treatment.

As always, WHO recommends that people who have cough, fever and difficulty breathing should seek medical care early. Patients should inform health care providers if they have travelled in the 14 days before they developed symptoms, or if they have been in close contact with someone who has been sick with respiratory symptoms.

(3) Wearing a medical mask can help limit the spread of some respiratory disease. However, using a mask alone is not guaranteed to stop infections and should be combined with other prevention measures including hand and respiratory hygiene and avoiding close contact— at least 1 metre (3 feet) distance between yourself and other people.

WHO advises on rational use of medical masks thus avoiding unnecessary wastage of precious resources and potential mis-use of masks (see "Advice on the Use of Masks"). This means using masks only if you have respiratory symptoms (coughing or sneezing), have suspected 2019-nCoV infection with mild symptoms or are caring for someone with suspected 2019-nCoV infection.

Advice on the
Use of Masks

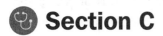 Section C

I Enhanced Learning【深度学习　以史为鉴】

A

The 1918 influenza pandemic was the most severe pandemic in recent history. It was caused by an H1N1 virus with genes of avian origin. Although there is not universal consensus regarding where the virus originated, it spread worldwide during 1918−1919. Mortality was high in people younger than 5 years old, 20−40 years old, and 65 years and older. The high mortality in healthy people, including those in the 20−40-year-age group, was a unique feature of this pandemic.

B

The Spanish flu pandemic of 1918, the deadliest in history, infected an estimated 500 million people worldwide—about one-third of the planet's population—and killed an estimated 20 million to 50 million victims, including some 675,000 Americans. The 1918 flu swiftly spread around the world, and bodies piled up in makeshift morgues before the virus ended its deadly global march.

C

The first wave of the 1918 pandemic occurred in the spring and was generally mild. The

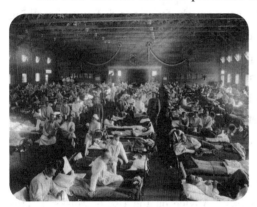

sick, who experienced such typical flu symptoms as chills, fever and fatigue, usually recovered after several days, and the number of reported deaths was low. However, a second, highly contagious wave of influenza appeared with a vengeance in the fall of that same year. Victims died within hours or days of developing symptoms, their skin turning blue and their lungs filling with fluid that caused them to suffocate. In just one year, 1918, the average life expectancy in America plummeted by a dozen years.

D

It's unknown exactly where the particular strain of influenza that caused the pandemic came from; however, the 1918 flu was first observed in Europe, America and areas of Asia before spreading to almost every other part of the planet within a matter of months. Despite the fact that the 1918 flu wasn't isolated to one place, it became known around the world as the Spanish flu, as Spain was hit hard by the disease and was not subject to the wartime news blackouts that affected other European countries. (Even Spain's king, Alfonso XIII reportedly contracted the flu.)

E

One unusual aspect of the 1918 flu was that it struck down many previously healthy, young people—a group normally resistant to this type of infectious illness—including a number of World War I servicemen. In fact, more U.S. soldiers died from the 1918 flu than were killed in battle during the war. Forty percent of the U.S. Navy was hit with the flu, while 36 percent of the Army became ill, and troops moving around the world in crowded ships and trains helped to spread the killer virus. Although the death toll attributed to the Spanish flu is often estimated at 20 million to 50 million victims worldwide, other estimates run as high as 100 million victims. The exact numbers are impossible to know due to a lack of medical record-keeping in many places.

F

When the 1918 flu hit, doctors and scientists were unsure what caused it or how to treat it. Unlike today, there were no effective vaccines or antiviral drugs that treat the flu. (The first licensed flu vaccine appeared in America in the 1940s. By the following decade, vaccine manufacturers could routinely produce vaccines that would help control and prevent future pandemics.) Complicating matters was the fact that World War Ⅰ had left parts of America with a shortage of physicians and other health workers. And of the available medical personnel in the U.S., many came down with the flu themselves. Additionally, hospitals in some areas were so overloaded with flu patients that schools, private homes and other buildings had to be converted into makeshift hospitals, some of which were staffed by medical students.

G

Officials in some communities imposed quarantines, ordered citizens to wear masks and shut down public places, including schools, churches and theaters. People were advised to avoid shaking hands and to stay indoors, libraries put a halt on lending books and regulations were passed banning spitting. According to *The New York Times*, during the pandemic, Boy Scouts in New York City approached people they'd seen spitting on the

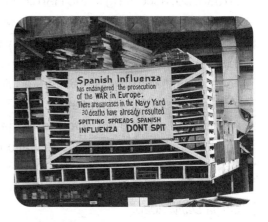

street and gave them cards that read: "You are in violation of the Sanitary Code."

H

The flu took a heavy human toll, wiping out entire families and leaving countless widows and orphans in its wake. Funeral parlors were overwhelmed and bodies piled up. Many people had to dig graves for their own family members. The flu was also detrimental to the economy. In the United States, businesses were forced to shut down because so many employees were sick. Basic services such as mail delivery and garbage collection were hindered due to flu-stricken workers. In some places there weren't enough farm workers to harvest crops. Even state and local health departments closed for business, hampering efforts to chronicle the spread of the 1918 flu and provide the public with answers about it.

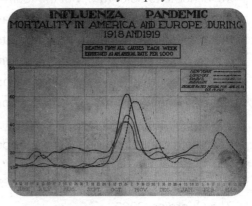

I

By the summer of 1919, the flu pandemic came to an end, as those that were infected either died or developed immunity. Almost 90 years later, in 2008, researchers announced they'd discovered what made the 1918 flu so deadly: A group of three genes enabled the virus to weaken a victim's bronchial tubes and lungs and clear the way for bacterial pneumonia.

(*Source:* CDC, March 20, 2019; History.com Editors, 31 January, 2020)

II Extensive Learning【拓展学习　媒体动态】

A pregnant woman infected with novel coronavirus gave birth to a healthy baby girl in a hospital in Harbin, capital of Northeast China's Heilongjiang province, on Jan. 30, according to the Harbin Municipal Health Commission on Monday.

According to the hospital, the baby weighed 3.05 kilograms and was given a 10 Apgar score at birth. When the 38-week pregnant woman was reported to the mission on Jan. 30, a group of obstetric, respiratory and neonatology experts gave her a consultation. To prevent the adult from getting worse, experts decided to do a cesarean section immediately.

All the medical workers involved in the operation have no occupational exposure and are now under isolation observation.

Read more from
China Daily, 2020

Read more 1-1

We don't yet know how dangerous the new coronavirus is, and we won't know until more data comes in. The 170 deaths from about 7,700 reported cases means the mortality rate is around 2%.

There were fears that the coronavirus might spread more widely during the week-long lunar new year holiday, which started on 24 January, when millions of Chinese travel home to celebrate, but the festivities have largely been cancelled and Wuhan and other cities in Hubei province are in lockdown. At the moment, it appears that people in poor health are at greatest risk, as is always the case with flu. A key concern is the range of severity of symptoms—some people appear to suffer only mild illness while others are becoming severely ill. This makes it more difficult to establish the true number of infected people and the extent of transmission. But the authorities are keen to stop the spread and anxious about whether the virus could become more potent than it so far appears to be.

Read more from
The Guardian, 2020

Read more 1-2

Pharmacies say they have seen a spike in sales of hand sanitisers and more demand for face masks in the wake of the coronavirus outbreak.

While virologists say hand sanitising can help stop the virus, they say there is not much evidence that face masks help.

Hand washing with soap is still the best cleaning practice, says the NHS.

Nonetheless, some online shops show a shortage of sanitiser and some stores are saying they don't stock masks.

Boots has seen an increase in sales of its own brand anti-viral hand foam and hand sanitisers, the BBC understands, and while some lines are out of stock, others can still be bought.

Read more from
BBC Business, 2020

Read more 1-3

A fifth novel coronavirus patient in Shanghai recovered from infection Wednesday, as 16 new cases were reported in the city on the same day, bringing the total confirmed cases to 96.

Wu Jinglei, director of Shanghai Municipal Health Commission, said at a press conference Wednesday Shanghai has expedited efforts across the city to battle the novel coronavirus and expanded the screening scope from medical institutions to roads, ports, airports, and communities, which ultimately led to the detection of 16 confirmed cases.

The city has started to report the number of cases of coronavirus infection every 12 hours, instead of the previous 24 hours.

Shanghai also launched an extended prescription and delivery service under which local residents can get prescriptions from the family doctors they sign up with and have their medicine delivered at their doorsteps. This will minimize the need for individuals to venture out.

Read more from
Global Times, 2020

Read more 1-4

Video Resources for Extensive Learning

（1）1918 Spanish flu pandemic.（Video1-2）

（2）Spanish flu: A warning from history.（Video1-3）

（3）Flu season: Three things to know.（Video1-4）

（4）Coronavirus: New global outbreaks.（Video1-5）

Video 1-2　Video 1-3

Video 1-4　Video 1-5

Section D

Projects in Practice【实践探索　行动项目】

1. Project 1

Matching Headings: There are ten short statements in this project. Each statement contains information given in one of the paragraphs of the passage in Section C Enhanced Learning. Read through the passage and identify the paragraph from which the information is derived. You may choose a paragraph more than once. Each paragraph is marked with a letter. Answer the questions by filling the corresponding letter in each blank below.

_____ (1) With no specific medicine against influenza infections, people were uncapable of getting rid of the flu.

_____ (2) The low mortality at the early epidemic stage may result from a soon recovery after infection.

_____ (3) Patients who recovered from the infection became immune to the flu, contributing to an end of the pandemic.

_____ (4) Over one third of the U.S. Army was infected.

_____ (5) Kids played an important role in maintaining the cleaning of the city.

_____ (6) Firms and companies were closed due to insufficient healthy labors.

_____ (7) Control efforts were limited to non-pharmaceutical interventions such as isolation, quarantine, and good personal hygiene.

_____ (8) After its early trace in Asia, the flu became viral worldwide.

_____ (9) About one billion people remained intact against the flu during the pandemic.

_____ (10) A higher risk of death of infected adults below forty, compared with the cases in other pandemics, is typical of the Spanish flu.

Key 1-1

2. Project 2

Viewpoint: Discuss with group members your reasons for the choices in Project 1, and then share your opinion on the topic "What College Students Can Do to Help Others During the Pandemic".

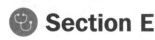 **Section E**

Self-assessment【进阶评估　自我超越】

1. Cooperative Learning Assessment

Please check your contribution to the group after the project is done.

	Superior (5)	Above Average (4)	Average (3)	Below Average (2)	Weak (1)
Understood what was required for the project					
Participated in the group discussion					
Helped the group to function well as a team					
Contributed useful ideas					
How much work was done					
Quality of completed work					
What could you improve upon next time?					
Your group members' comments					
Your group leader's comments					

2. Assessment of Individual Study

Instructions:

(1) Read each statement in the table below and place a check mark in the column that best describes how well you can complete that task.

(2) Review your responses for each task. If you have checked five or more in the "Somewhat" and / or "No" columns, you may need to consider making greater efforts after class.

I can	Yes	Somewhat	No
Understand the main idea of the text			
Identify the major points, important facts and details, and vocabulary in the text			
Make inferences about what is implied in the text			
Recognize the organization and purpose of the text			
Remember the new words and expressions			
Speak on the topic effectively			
Employ search strategy to gain information to address the project			
Refer to appropriate resources to deal with the project			

3. Personal Development

Instruction:

Completing this section will help you make informed practicing decisions. Please identify your strengths, and the areas that you need to develop or strengthen and record them below.

STRENGTHS:
I am confident that I can...
(1)
(2)
(3)
AREAS FOR IMPROVEMENT:
I would like to improve my ability to...
(1)
(2)
(3)

Unit 2　First Aid Treatment

院前急救

Section A

Warm-up Activity【敬佑生命　仁爱健康】

Try to serve as a first aider with your group members based upon the video "What to Do During an Earthquake-emergency Preparedness"（Video1–6）and "First Aid in Seizures"（Video1–7）.

Here is an example:

What is to be done for better emergency preparedness?

(1)　What to do during an earthquake-emergency preparedness.

(2)　First aid in seizures.

Video 1–6

Video 1–7

More Prepared Minutes

Emergency Preparedness Kits (锦囊) to reduce injury (受伤) and increase chances of your survival (幸存) during an earthquake and seizure attack are provided as following.

Emergency survival experts agree: "Drop, Cover, and Hold on" is your best plan during an earthquake to save your life. If you are indoors, stay there, drop to the ground, cover your head and neck with your hands and arms. Avoid exterior walls (外墙), windows, heavy furniture (家具), fire places and more appliances (电器). The kitchen is a very dangerous place. If you are outdoors, get into the open, stay clear of buildings, power lines, trees, or anything else that will fall on you. Do not stand in a doorway. Do not be close to exterior walls that will probably collapse (倒塌) firstly.

And how to give emergency medical aid to seizure (癫痫) patients may be recommended. Relax, pass-by move back! Move any potentially harmful objects out of harm's way to prevent injury. Don't restrain (限制) him or her from moving, provide head support and wait for the attack to end. After seizure attack eases (缓解), move the patient onto the side and tilt his or her head back to protect against choking (窒息) from possible vomiting (呕吐).

Section B

Ⅰ First Aid【救死扶伤　生命至上】

1. Casualty (意外受伤)

Call a doctor or ambulance (救护车) awaiting professional (专业的) medical assistance. If the casualty is conscious (有意识的), ask if there is any pain, and if so where. Look for signs of injury as bleeding (流血), swelling (肿胀), deformity (破损), or signs of illness as a raised temperature and irregular pulse (脉搏异常) etc. Look inside the lips for any trace of blueness which might indicate asphyxia (窒息). Loosen clothing around the neck to facilitate (促进) breathing. All treatment, either through emergency resuscitation or by controlling shock, is to sustain (维持) life. To prevent the condition worsening, wounds should be covered, injured areas should be immobilized (固定), casualty should not be removed. Relate (陈述) all of the above information to the qualified (专业的) first aider on his arrival.

2. Cardiac Arrest (心脏骤停)

Sudden cardiac arrest can happen to anyone, at any time. With AED and CPR training, you can learn how to save a life when every moment counts. You can learn when-and-how to use an emergency procedure (CRP) and an automated external defibrillator (AED). When should an AED and CRP be used? CPR is a very important action for saving a patient's life. However, an AED is crucial (重要的) towards regaining the natural rhythm of the heartbeat as well as restarting the patient's heart.

CPR, or cardiopulmonary resuscitation, is an emergency procedure to assist someone who has suffered cardiac arrest. An emergency procedure consists of (由……组成) external cardiac massage (心脏按压) and artificial respiration (人工呼吸); the first treatment for a person who has collapsed and has no pulse and has stopped breathing; attempts to restore circulation (恢复循环) of the blood and prevent death or brain damage due to lack of oxygen.

AED, or automated external defibrillator is a portable electronic device (携便式电子设备) that automatically diagnoses (自动诊断) the life-threatening cardiac arrest. The Lifeline AED is also a semi-automatic defibrillator (半自动除颤器) that is technologically advanced enough to include all mission critical features necessary to provide the most advanced treatment for Sudden Cardiac Arrest.

3. Video Learning

Learn CPR and AED procedures.（Video1-8）

Video 1-8

Ⅱ Notes【说文解字　名词注释】

1. Vocabulary Table

Vocabulary 1-2

Words & Expressions	Part of Speech	Meaning in Text
kit	*n.*	锦囊
injury	*n.*	受伤
survival	*n.*	生存；幸存
exterior wall	*phr.*	外墙
furniture	*n.*	家具
appliance	*n.*	电器
collapse	*vt.*	倒塌
seizure	*n.*	癫痫
restrain	*vt.*	限制
ease	*vt.*	缓解
choke	*vt.*	窒息
vomite	*vt.*	呕吐
casualty	*n.*	意外受伤；伤者
ambulance	*n.*	救护车
professional	*adj.*	专业的
conscious	*phr.*	有意识的
bleeding	*vt.*	流血
swelling	*vt.*	肿胀
deformity	*n.*	破损
irregular pulse	*phr.*	脉搏异常
asphyxia	*n.*	窒息
facilitate	*vt.*	促进
sustain	*vt.*	维持
immobilize	*vt.*	固定
relate to	*phr.*	向……陈述
qualified	*adj.*	专业的
cardiac arrest	*phr.*	心脏骤停
crucial	*adj.*	重要的；关键的
consist of	*phr.*	由……组成
cardiac massage	*phr.*	心脏按压
artificial respiration	*phr.*	人工呼吸
restore circulation	*phr.*	恢复循环
portable electronic device	*phr.*	便携式电子设备
automatically diagnoses	*phr.*	自动诊断
semi-automatic defibrillator	*phr.*	半自动除颤器

2. Useful Knowledge

(1) bleeding, swelling, deformity or signs of illness as a raised temperature：流血、肿胀、破损和体温升高等征兆。

(2) the lips for any trace of blueness which might indicate asphyxia：嘴唇是否呈紫色以辨别会否窒息。

(3) Cardiopulmonary Resuscitation (CPR)：心肺复苏术。

心肺复苏 (CPR)是针对呼吸、心跳停止的急症危重病人所采取的关键抢救措施,即胸外按压形成暂时的人工循环并恢复自主搏动,采用人工呼吸代替自主呼吸,快速电除颤转复心室颤动,以及尽早使用血管活性药物来重新恢复自主循环的急救技术。

(4) Automated External Defibrillator (AED)：自动体外除颤器。

自动体外除颤器是由普通人操作的对发生心室纤颤患者进行电击除颤的先进设备。大部分CA发生在院外,部分人CA发作前会有先兆,及早识别CA发作,发作时第一反应者及时实施CPR,获得自动体外除颤仪 (AED) 及时除颤,当地有高效、专业的急诊医疗服务体系(EMSS) 是决定患者存活的关键。此类急救设备的设置,代表一个城市的安全和文明发展程度。自动体外除颤器 (AED) 在抢救心脏骤停患者方面效果显著,被称为"救命神器"。

3. Idiomatic Usage

(1) professional medical assistance：专业医护援助。

(2) signs of injury：伤情。

(3) irregular pulse：脉搏异常。

(4) qualified first aider：专业急救员。

(5) to prevent the condition worsening：防止伤情恶化。

(6) emergency resuscitation：心肺复苏。

(7) cardiac arrest：心脏停搏；心脏骤停。

(8) artificial respiration：人工呼吸。

(9) brain damage：脑损伤。

(10) due to：由于；应付。

(11) lack of：缺少；缺乏。

4. English-Chinese Translation

(1) First aid for casualty.（Resource 1-1）

(2) First aid in cardiac arrest.（Resource 1-1）

Resource 1-1

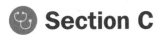 Section C

Ⅰ Enhanced Learning【深度学习　健康关爱】

First aid steps in the right order:

(　　) If the casualty is conscious, ask if there is any pain, and if so where.

(　　) Loosen clothing around the neck to facilitate breathing.

(　　) Look for signs of injury as bleeding, swelling or signs of illness as a raised temperature and irregular pulse etc.

(　　) Look inside the lips for any trace of blueness which might indicate asphyxia.

(　　) All treatment, either through emergency resuscitation or controlling shock, is to sustain life.

(　　) To prevent the condition worsening, wounds should be covered, injured areas should be immobilized, casualty should not be removed.

(　　) Call a doctor or ambulance awaiting professional medical assistance.

(　　) Relate all of the above information to the qualified first aider on his arrival.

Key 1-2

Ⅱ Extensive Learning【拓展学习　媒体动态】

Seven Ways to Improve Your Lung Capacity

Do Breathing Exercises

Take a deep breath. No, really, it is that simple. There are a number of breathing exercises you can do that help keep your lungs healthy. One involves standing up with your back arched (成弓形弯曲的), breathing in and holding your breath for 10 seconds before exhaling (呼气) — which can easily be done while watching the TV.

Consume Enough Vitamin D

A study released this year found that higher vitamin D levels were associated with (与……有关) better lung function (肺功能). In the summer, depending on where you live, most people can get enough vitamin D from the sunshine. As the winter months approach (来临) and the sun disappears, it may be worth investing in vitamin D supplements (补充; 添加). Vitamin D can also be found in foods such as oily fish, egg yolks (蛋黄) and red meat.

Indulge Your Inner Musician

If you are one of the many people who enjoy singing in the shower then you may be in luck, because singing can, apparently, aid lung capacity (肺活量). According to the British Lung Foundation, it's particularly helpful for patients with respiratory diseases (呼吸道疾病). People with lung conditions told the foundation that controlling their breathing through singing helped manage their conditions. It is an area that is still being investigated. A study of 20 Indonesian students, published in 2015, found that the average (平均的) lung capacity of choir singers was higher than that of non-singers.

Sort out Your Posture

Studies have shown that slumped (倒下的) sitting decreases (降低) lung capacity, because the position squeezes (挤压) your lungs, making them smaller. So, for a very quick fix, sit up straight to get the best lung capacity you can. A good posture (姿势) can help with back pain, too.

Video Resources for Extensive Learning

（1）First aid treatments—how to do CPR.（Video 1-9）

（2）What does an AED do?（Video 1-10）

Video 1-9

Video 1-10

Section D

Projects in Practice【实践探索　行动项目】

1. Project 1

Situational Interaction

Watch the following video（Video 1-11）and discuss within your group how to help a choking person as quickly as possible.

Video 1-11

2. Project 2

Situational Play:Video-based Practice

(1) CPR simple steps to save a life.（Video 1-12）

(2) AED plus rescue.（Video 1-13）

Video 1-12

Video 1-13

Section E

Self-assessment【进阶评估　自我超越】

1. Cooperative Learning Assessment

Please check your contribution to the group after the project is done.

	Superior (5)	Above Average (4)	Average (3)	Below Average (2)	Weak (1)
Understood what was required for the project					
Participated in the group discussion					
Helped the group to function well as a team					
Contributed useful ideas					
How much work was done					
Quality of completed work					
What could you improve upon next time?					
Your group members' comments					
Your group leader's comments					

2. Assessment of Your Study

Instructions:

(1) Read each statement in the table below and place a check mark in the column that best describes how well you can complete that task.

(2) Review your responses for each task. If you have checked five or more in the "Somewhat" and / or "No" columns, you may need to consider making greater efforts after class.

I can	Yes	Somewhat	No
Understand the main idea of the text			
Identify the major points, important facts and details, and vocabulary in the text			
Make inferences about what is implied in the text			
Recognize the organization and purpose of the text			
Remember the new words and expressions			
Speak on the topic effectively			
Employ search strategy to gain information to address the project			
Refer to appropriate resources to deal with the project			

3. Say What You Want to Say

Please start what you want to say.（Resource 1-2）

Resource 1-2

Unit 3　Diet and Nutrition

膳食营养

Section A

Warm-up Activity【健康膳食　灿烂明天】

Try to serve as a dietician with your group members based upon the video from "kitchen stories".

1. Practice Easy 10 Breakfast Recipe（Video1-14）

2. Crock-pot Express Crock Multi-cooker Review and Demo（Video1-15）

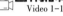

Video 1-14

Section B

Ⅰ Healthy Dining Habits【餐饮习惯　健康向上】

Video 1-15

1. Cooking Tips（建议）

(1) Eat what's in season.

Visit farmer's markets when you can, and use what's in season for optimal (最佳的) taste.

(2) Add citrus fruits (柑橘类水果) for contrast.

To bring out the zing in everything from fish to meat, add juice from lemons, oranges, or grapefruits.

(3) Stock up on stock.

Stock is "the flavor foundation of French cuisine". It's best if you can make your own; then use it as a umami base for all your sauces and soups (汤).

(4) Make sea salt a staple.

Fine sea salt is a standard (标准) for seasoning all dishes.

2. Keep a Healthy Diet (饮食)

(1) Charred meat.

Charred meat often contains pro-inflammatory hydrocarbons. That's no good since inflammation can break down your skin's precious collagen.

(2) Alcohol.

The effects of alcohol (酒) on your liver are harmful. If toxins build up in your liver, and aren't broken down properly, your skin can develop a variety of issues (各种各样问题).

(3) Salty foods.

Excess (过剩的) salt in the body draws more fluid (液体) out of the cells (细胞) to help neutralize (抵销) the salt and draw it out of the body. As a result, your skin gets drier because of the lack of fluid.

(4) Anything super spicy.

Spicy (辛辣的) foods trigger inflammation and flushing (炎症).

3. Diet Tips

Chinese Breakfast / 中式早餐

Main Course **主盘**	congee	粥
	soybean milk	豆浆
	fried noodles	炒面
	boiled egg	煮鸡蛋
	steamed bun	馒头
	fried egg	炒蛋
	noodle soup	汤面
	won ton	云吞 / 馄饨
	deep-fried twisted dough	油条
Teas &Drinks **茶类及饮料**	oolong tea	乌龙茶
	milk	牛奶
	coffee	咖啡

Chinese Lunch / 中式午餐

Chinese Dishes **中式菜谱**	roast duck	烤鸭
	hot pot	火锅
	abalone	鲍鱼
	sea cucumber	海参
	cashew chicken	腰果鸡丁
	shark's fin soup	鱼翅汤
	grouper	石斑鱼
	sautéed prawns	炸明虾
	celery	芹菜
	crab	螃蟹
	fish balls	鱼丸
	lobster	龙虾
	shrimp	虾
	roast pig	烤乳猪
	Chinese mushroom	香菇
	hair vegetables	发菜
	lotus root	莲藕
	scallop	干贝

Chinese Dishes 中式菜谱	sweet and sour pork	糖醋排骨
	rice wine	米酒
	steamed rice	米饭
	pork dumplings	猪肉饺子

Chinese Dinner / 中式晚餐

Chinese Dishes 中式菜谱	almond junket	杏仁豆腐
	jellyfish	海蜇
	barbecued pork buns	叉烧包
	mustard	芥末
	bean vermicelli	粉丝
	oyster saucer	耗油
	shrimp omelet	虾仁炒蛋
	Chinese ham	中国火腿
	steamed open dumplings	烧卖
	Chinese sausage	腊肠
	custard tart	蛋挞
	won ton	云吞 / 馄饨
	spring rolls	春卷
	sweet soup balls	汤圆
	spare ribs	排骨
	red bean dessert	红豆汤
	steamed rice	米饭
	stuffed dumplings	饺子

Western Breakfast/西式早餐

Fresh Squeezed 鲜榨果汁	orange	橙汁
	carrot	胡萝卜汁
	grapefruit	西柚汁
	seasonal juice of the day	当日时令鲜榨果汁
Fresh Eggs 新鲜鸡蛋	poached	水波蛋
	easy over	双面煎蛋
	boiled	煮鸡蛋
	scrambled	炒蛋
	sunny-side up	单面煎蛋
Food 美食	toasted bread	各色吐司
	bacon	熏猪肉
	pork sausages	猪肉肠
	potatoes and tomatoes	土豆和西红柿

Drinks 饮料	fresh brewed coffee with cream	现磨咖啡配奶油
	decaffeinated coffee with milk	无咖啡因咖啡配牛奶
Teas 茶类 with... 配……	English tea	英国红茶
	green tea	绿茶
	jasmine tea	茉莉花茶
	with lemon	配柠檬
	with milk	配牛奶
	with ceam	配奶油

Western Lunch / 西式午餐

Vegetables Salad 蔬菜色拉	lettuce	莴苣
	tomato	西红柿
	onion	洋葱
	mashed potato	土豆泥
	with French dressing	配法式调味酱
Main Course 主盘	apple pie	苹果馅饼
	chicken nugget	炸鸡块
	hamburger	汉堡
	French fries	炸薯条
	hot dog	热狗
	pizza	比萨
	sandwich	三明治
	sausage	香肠
	doughnut	炸面团
Desserts 甜点	biscuits	甜饼干
	cream	奶油
	ice-cream	冰激凌
	milk shake	奶昔
	chocolate cake	巧克力蛋糕
	lemonade	柠檬水

Western Dinner / 西式晚餐

Salad 沙拉	salad	色拉
Main Course 主盘	baked potato	烤土豆
	corn-on-the-cob	玉米棒
	fish pie	鱼馅饼
	meatballs	肉丸
	roast beef	烤牛肉
	steak	牛排
	soup	汤

	pork chop	猪排
Main Course 主盘	mutton chop	羊排
	spaghetti	意大利面条
	roast chicken	烤鸡
Desserts 甜点	chocolate pudding	巧克力布丁
	cheese	奶酪
	crackers	饼干
	cake	蛋糕
Wine & Drinks 酒及饮料	red wine	红酒
	beer	啤酒
	coffee	咖啡

Ⅱ Notes【说文解字　名词注释】

1. Vocabulary Table

Vocabulary 1–3

Words & Expressions	Part of Speech	Meaning in Text
tip	*n.*	建议
optimal	*adj.*	最佳的
citrus fruits	*phr.*	柑橘类水果
soup	*n.*	汤
standard	*n.*	标准
diet	*n.*	饮食
alcohol	*n.*	酒
a variety of issues	*phr.*	各种各样的问题
excess	*adj.*	过剩的
fluid	*n.*	液体
cell	*n.*	细胞
neutralize	*vt.*	抵销
spicy	*adj.*	辛辣的
inflammation	*n.*	炎症

2. Useful Knowledge

(1) use what's in season for optimal taste：使用应季食材能做出最美的味道。

(2) add citrus for contrast：加点柑橘类让味道不一样。

(3) to bring out the zing in everything from fish to meat：为了让鱼肉和其他肉的味道鲜美。

(4) "Stock is 'the flavor foundation of French cuisine'."的意思是：高汤是"法国菜的风味担当"。

(5) a standard for seasoning all dishes：所有菜调味的必需品。

(6) The effects of alcohol on your liver are harmful：酒对肝脏会造成损害。

(7) "Excess salt in the body draws more fluid out of the cells."的意思是:体内盐分过量会从细胞内吸走更多的水分。

(8) "Spicy foods trigger inflammation and flushing."的意思是:辛辣食物会诱发炎症和脸红。

3. Idiomatic Usage

(1) cooking tips:厨房小贴士。

(2) keep a healthy diet:健康膳食。

(3) stock up on stock:存点高汤。

(4) make sea salt a staple:主要用海盐。

(5) build up:堆积。

(6) break down:分解。

(7) as a result:结果。

(8) It's no good (use) doing sth.:做某事毫无益处。

4. English-Chinese Translation

(1) Cooking tips.(Resource 1–3)

(2) Keep a healthy diet.(Resource 1–3)

Resource 1–3

Section C

Ⅰ Enhanced Learning【深度学习　膳食均衡】

Matching Game

(　　)(1) 吃应季食物　　　　　a. for optimal taste

(　　)(2) 最美的味道　　　　　b. stock up on stock

(　　)(3) 存点高汤　　　　　　c. make sea salt a staple

(　　)(4) 各种各样问题　　　　d. seasoning all dishes

(　　)(5) 主要用海盐　　　　　e. eat what's in season

(　　)(6) 调味品菜　　　　　　f. a variety of issues

(　　)(7) 体内过多的盐分　　　g. excess salt in the body

(　　)(8) 酒对肝脏是有害的　　h. alcohol on your liver are harmful

Key 1–3

Ⅱ Extensive Learning【拓展学习　媒体动态】

Diets Add Years to Your Life As Well As Help Lose Weight

New research suggests that people who use the trendy new diets that involve intermittent (间歇的) fasting may actually be adding years to their lives. It turns out the celebrities promoting the lifestyle, like Kourtney Kardashian and Jennifer Aniston, may actually be onto (到……之上)

something.

There are several types of intermittent fasting diets, but most involve either limiting food intake to just an 8-hour window or not eating for two days a week.

Professor Mark Mattson, a neuroscientist (神经科学家), has studied the effects of the diet for over two decades (and has been practicing it himself for 20 years).

"We are at a transition point where we could soon consider adding information about intermittent fasting to medical school curricula alongside standard advice about healthy diets and exercise," Mattson told SWNS.

His findings, which were published in the New England Journal of Medicine, show that fasting can trigger "metabolic switching (新陈代谢)", and evolutionary (进化的) adaption. Studies show that aside from helping with metabolism, fasting has also been linked with decreased blood pressure, cholesterol (胆固醇) and resting heart rates. It may also help control blood sugar levels, increase resistance (抵抗力) to stress and suppress (镇压) inflammation (炎症).

Of course, intermittent fasting has its downside as well.

(*Source*: Fox News, Dec. 2019)

Video Resources for Extensive Learning
The traditional Chinese medicine diet.（Video 1–16）

Video 1–16

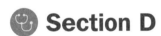 **Section D**

Projects in Practice【实践探索　行动项目】

1. Project 1
Situational Interaction
Discuss within your group how to practice "Meals Serving List" as clear as possible.

**Meals Serving List
餐饮工作单 (西式早餐)**

TO / 至: Mary（housekeeper, 家政服务员）
FROM / 由: Mr. Smith（host, 主人）
SUBJECT / 主题: Meals Serving 餐饮服务
DATE / 日期:＿＿＿＿＿＿＿月 / 日

Message / 正文：

Please do some serving, following what I ticked out in the serving list.

Thanks！(请参照餐单上所✓的项提供相关服务，谢谢！)

Fresh Squeezed 鲜榨果汁	☐Orange 橙汁 ☐Grapefruit 西柚汁	☐Carrot 胡萝卜 ☐Seasonal Juice of the Day 当日时令鲜榨果汁
Fresh Eggs 新鲜鸡蛋	☐Poached 水波蛋 ☐Boiled 煮鸡蛋 ☐Sunny-side Up 单面煎蛋	☐Easy Over 双面煎蛋 ☐Scrambled 炒蛋
Food 美食	☐Toasted Bread 各色吐司 ☐Pork Sausages 猪肉肠	☐Bacon 熏猪肉 ☐Potatoes and Tomatoes 土豆 / 西红柿
Drinks 饮料	☐Fresh Brewed Coffee with Cream 现磨咖啡配奶油 ☐Decaffeinated Coffee with Milk 无咖啡因咖啡配牛奶	
Teas 茶类 with ... 配……	With 配	☐English 英国红茶 ☐Jasmine 茉莉花茶 ☐Green 绿茶 ☐Lemon 柠檬 ☐Milk 牛奶 ☐Cream 奶油

Meals Serving List
餐饮工作单 (西式中餐)

TO / 至: Mary（housekeeper，家政服务员）

FROM / 由: Mr. Smith（host，主人）

SUBJECT / 主题: Meals Serving 餐饮服务

DATE / 日期：＿＿＿＿＿＿＿月 /日

Message / 正文：

Please do some serving, following what I ticked out in the serving list.

Thanks! (请参照餐单上所✓的项提供相关服务，谢谢！)

Vegetables Salad 蔬菜色拉	☐Lettuce	莴苣
	☐Tomato	西红柿
	☐Onion	洋葱
	☐Mashed Potato	土豆泥
	☐With French Dressing	配法式调味酱
Main Course 主盘	☐Apple Pie	苹果馅饼
	☐Chicken Nugget	炸鸡块
	☐Hamburger	汉堡
	☐French Fries	炸薯条
	☐Hot Dog	热狗
	☐Pizza	比萨
	☐Sandwich	三明治

Main Course 主盘	□Sausage	香肠
	□Doughnut	炸面团
Desserts 甜点	□Biscuits	甜饼干
	□Cream	奶油
	□Ice-cream	冰激凌
	□Milk Shake	奶昔
	□Chacolate Cake	巧克力蛋糕
	□Lemonade	柠檬水

Meals Serving List
餐饮工作单 (西式晚餐)

TO / 至: Mary（housekeeper，家政服务员）

FROM / 由: Mr. Smith（host，主人）

SUBJECT / 主题: Meals Serving 餐饮服务

DATE / 日期:＿＿＿＿＿＿＿月/日

Message / 正文:

Please do some serving, following what I ticked out in the serving list.

Thanks!

(请参照餐单上所√的项提供相关服务，谢谢！)

Salad 色拉	□Salad	色拉
Main Course 主盘	□Baked Potapo	烤土豆
	□Fish Pie	鱼馅饼
	□Meatballs	肉丸
	□Roast Beef	烤牛肉
	□Soup	汤
	□Roast Chicken	烤鸡
	□Spaghetti	意大利面
	□Corn-on-the-cob	玉米棒
	□Steak	牛排
	□Pizza	比萨
	□Pork Chop	猪排
Desserts 甜点	□Chocolate Pudding	巧克力布丁
	□Cheese	奶酪
	□Cake	蛋糕
	□Milk Shake	奶昔
	□Lemonade	柠檬水
Wine&Drinks 酒水	□Red Wine	红酒
	□Beer	啤酒
	□Coffee	咖啡

2. Project 2

Situational Play:Video-based Practice

(1) Learn useful formal table setting in English with pictures.（Video 1-17）

(2) How to make a full English breakfast.（Video 1-18）

Video 1-17

Video 1-18

 Section E

Self-assesment【进阶评估　自我超越】

1. Cooperative Learning Assessment

Please check your contribution to the group after the project is done.

	Superior (5)	Above Average (4)	Average (3)	Below Average (2)	Weak (1)
Understood what was required for the project					
Participated in the group discussion					
Helped the group to function well as a team					
Contributed useful ideas					
How much work was done					
Quality of completed work					
What could you improve upon next time?					
Your group members' comments					
Your group leader's comments					

2. Assessment of Your Study

Instructions:

(1) Read each statement in the table below and place a check mark in the column that best describes how well you can complete that task.

(2) Review your responses for each task. If you have checked five or more in the "Somewhat" and / or "No" columns, you may need to consider making greater efforts after class.

I can	Yes	Somewhat	No
Understand the main idea of the text			
Identify the major points, important facts and details, and vocabulary in the text			
Make inferences about what is implied in the text			
Recognize the organization and purpose of the text			
Remember the new words and expressions			
Speak on the topic effectively			
Employ search strategy to gain information to address the project			
Refer to appropriate resources to deal with the project			

3. Say What You Want to Say

Please start what you want to say.（Resource 1−4）

Resource 1−4

Chapter 2

Domestic Service

如数家"珍"

Unit 1　Garbage Sorting

垃圾分类

🩺 Section A

Warm-up Activity【地球环保　人人有责】

1. Read the Signs and Understand the Meaning Behind

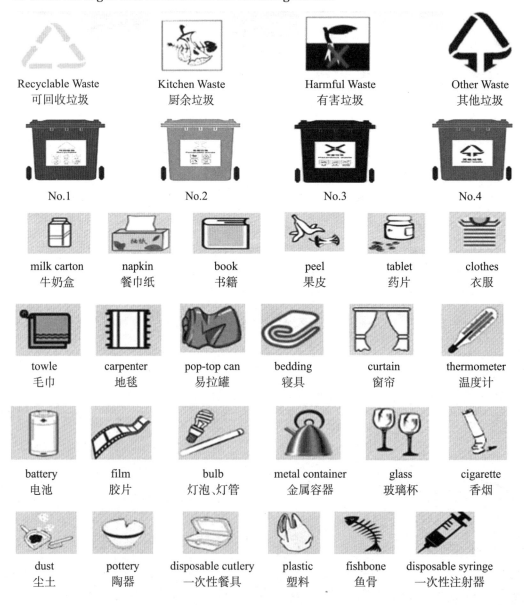

| Recyclable Waste 可回收垃圾 | Kitchen Waste 厨余垃圾 | Harmful Waste 有害垃圾 | Other Waste 其他垃圾 |

| No.1 | No.2 | No.3 | No.4 |

| milk carton 牛奶盒 | napkin 餐巾纸 | book 书籍 | peel 果皮 | tablet 药片 | clothes 衣服 |

| towle 毛巾 | carpenter 地毯 | pop-top can 易拉罐 | bedding 寝具 | curtain 窗帘 | thermometer 温度计 |

| battery 电池 | film 胶片 | bulb 灯泡、灯管 | metal container 金属容器 | glass 玻璃杯 | cigarette 香烟 |

| dust 尘土 | pottery 陶器 | disposable cutlery 一次性餐具 | plastic 塑料 | fishbone 鱼骨 | disposable syringe 一次性注射器 |

⚕ Section B

Video 2-1

Ⅰ Garbage Sorting【垃圾分类　从我做起】

1. Sorting Significance

Chinese President Xi Jinping has underlined efforts to cultivate (培养) the good habit of garbage classification to improve the living environment and contribute to green and sustainable (可持续的) development.

"Garbage classification is related to the people's living environment and the economical (节约的; 经济的) use of resources. It is also an important embodiment of the level of civic-mindedness (公民意识)," Xi said.

The key to carrying out waste sorting is to strengthen scientific management, form a mechanism (机制) with lasting effects, and cultivate the habit of waste sorting, Xi said, adding that China should strengthen guidance, adapt (采取) measures to local conditions, and make continuous, detailed and concrete efforts.

Through effective supervision (监管) and guidance, the country will let more people take action and cultivate the good habit of garbage classification to improve the living environment and contribute to green and sustainable development, Xi said.

"Lucid waters and lush mountains are invaluable assets. Extensive education and guidance should be carried out to make the people realize the importance and necessity of garbage sorting," Xi said.

By the end of 2020, garbage sorting systems will have been built in 46 major Chinese cities, and all cities at the prefecture (行政区域) level and above should have built such systems by 2025.

2. Regulation in Shanghai

According to the regulation (条例; 规则) in Shanghai China, people are required to sort household garbage (垃圾) into four categories—dry garbage, wet garbage (kitchen waste), recyclables and hazardous waste-and individuals (个人) who fail to do so will be fined (罚款) up to 200 yuan. For companies and institutions, the fine can go up to 50,000 yuan. In addition, transport operators can refuse to pick up the garbage if it's not properly sorted.

According to the regulation, if not requested by guests, hotels should not provide disposable (一次性的) slippers and shower caps, while restaurants and food delivery businesses should not provide disposable cutlery.

Government and public institutions are not allowed to use disposable cups in the office and should give priority (优先) in purchasing products made from recycled (可回收利用的) materials.

All the courier companies that operate in the city should use digital order (电子订单) and environment-friendly materials for packaging.

3. Dry or Wet Garbage

According to the regulation, people are required to sort household garbage into four categories—dry garbage, wet garbage (kitchen waste), recyclables and hazardous waste—and individuals who fail to do so will be fined up to 200 yuan. For companies and institutions, the fine can go up to 50,000 yuan. In addition, transport operators can refuse to pick up the garbage if it's not properly sorted.

II Notes【说文解字　名词注释】

🎧 Vocabulary 2–1

1. Vocabulary Table

Words & Expressions	Part of Speech	Meaning in Text
recyclable waste	*phr.*	可回收垃圾
kitchen waste	*phr.*	厨余垃圾
harmful waste	*phr.*	有害垃圾
other waste	*phr.*	其他垃圾
milk carton	*phr.*	牛奶盒
napkin	*n.*	餐巾纸
book	*n.*	书籍
peel	*n.*	果皮
tablet	*n.*	药片
clothes	*n.*	衣服
towel	*n.*	毛巾
carpenter	*n.*	地毯
pop-top can	*phr.*	易拉罐
bedding	*n.*	寝具
curtain	*n.*	窗帘
thermometer	*n.*	温度计
battery	*n.*	电池
film	*n.*	胶片
bulb	*n.*	灯泡;灯管
metal container	*phr.*	金属容器
glass	*n.*	玻璃杯
cigarette	*n.*	香烟
dust	*n.*	尘土
pottery	*n.*	陶器
plastic	*n.*	塑料
disposable cutlery	*phr.*	一次性餐具
fishbone	*n.*	鱼骨
disposable syringe	*phr.*	一次性注射器
regulation	*n.*	条例;规则

Words & Expressions	Part of Speech	Meaning in Text
garbage	*n.*	垃圾
individual	*n.*	个人
fine	*vt.*	罚款
disposable	*adj.*	一次性的
priority	*n.*	优先
recycled	*adj.*	可回收利用的
digital	*adj.*	数码电子的
cultivate	*vt.*	培养
sustainable	*adj.*	可持续的
economical	*adj.*	经济的;节约的
civic-mindedness	*n.*	公民意识
mechanism	*n.*	机制
adapt	*vt.*	采取
supervision	*n.*	监管
prefecture	*n.*	行政区域

2. Useful Knowledge

(1) garbage、rubbish、trash 和 waste 在英语里都有"垃圾、废物"意思,它们的区别在于在哪个国家更常用:

① garbage 是垃圾的美式英语说法。

② rubbish 是英式英语中垃圾的意思。

③ trash 也是美式英语中垃圾的意思,也可以用来指不值得尊重的人。

④ waste 是一个正式用语,指没有利用价值的东西,包括废品、垃圾、废物、废料或者指时间、金钱、精力等的浪费。

(2) cultivate the good habit of garbage classification: 培养垃圾分类的好习惯。

(3) green and sustainable development: 绿色和可持续发展。

(4) be related to the people's living environment and the economical use of resources:关系广大人民群众生活环境,关系节约使用资源。

(5) form a mechanism with lasting effects, and cultivate the habit of waste sorting:形成长效机制、推动习惯养成。

(6) make continuous, detailed and concrete efforts:把工作做细做实,持之以恒抓下去。

(7) "Lucid waters and lush mountains are invaluable assets."的意思是:绿水青山就是金山银山。

3. Idiomatic Usage

(1) 干/湿垃圾(厨余垃圾)/可回收/有害垃圾:dry / wet garbage (kitchen waste) / recyclables / hazardous waste。

(2) 垃圾分类:garbage classification / sorting。

(3) 一次性餐具(拖鞋、浴帽):disposable cutlery (slippers and shower caps)。

(4) 环保材料:environment-friendly materials。

(5) 可回收材料:recycled materials。

(6) 可再生资源:renewable resources。

(7) 可持续发展:sustainable development。

(8) 无废城市:zero-waste cities / no-waste cities / waste-free cities。

(9) 固体废物:solid waste。

(10) 生活垃圾:domestic garbage。

4. Background Information

(1) 2019年6月5日世界环境日到来之际,习近平作出重要指示强调,推行垃圾分类,关键是要加强科学管理、形成长效机制、推动习惯养成。

(2)《上海市生活垃圾管理条例》于2019年7月1日起施行。除了居民个人垃圾分类要求外,条例针对特定对象提出了强制性要求。对于网上盛传的小龙虾到底是干垃圾还是湿垃圾,《上海市生活垃圾分类投放指引》明确列举,"水产及其加工食品(鱼、鱼鳞、虾、虾壳、鱿鱼)"都归属于湿垃圾。

(3) 据报道现在有上门代收垃圾服务 (garbage pick-up service) 了,市民在出门前将打好包的垃圾放在家门口 (place their bagged household garbage at doorstep),每天上午定时会有专人负责拿走,每次服务支付1元人民币的费用。

(4)"你是什么垃圾?"等一语双关的表达很快也被外媒捕捉到了。全世界都在围观中国上海人。

5. English-Chinese Translation

(1) Garbage sorting.(Resource 2-1)

(2) Dry or wet garbage.(Resource 2-2)

Resource 2-1

Resource 2-2

Section C

Ⅰ Enhanced Learning【深度学习 放眼全球】

Read the text "Regulation in Shanghai" and complete the following passages.

根据《上海市生活垃圾管理条例》规定,人们须将家中的垃圾按照干垃圾、湿垃圾(厨余垃圾)、可回收物以及有害垃圾这四个类别放置,如果个人没有将垃圾分类投放最高罚款_____元人民币,单位混装混运最高罚款_____万元人民币。此外,_____的垃圾,收运单位可以拒绝接收。

条例规定,旅馆不得主动提供拖鞋、浴帽等一次性日用品,餐饮服务提供者和餐饮配送服务提供者不得主动提供一次性餐具。

党政机关、事业单位内部办公场所不得使用,采购时应优先选择由_____制成的产品。

上海所有快递企业都应使用_____包装。

Key 2-1

Ⅱ Extensive Learning【拓展学习　媒体动态】

Garbage Classification in Different Countries

重点要告知的是乱丢垃圾在美国是一种犯罪行为！美国各州都有禁止乱扔垃圾的法律，乱丢杂物属三级轻罪，可处以300到1000美元不等的罚款、入狱或社区服务（最长一年），也可以上述两种或三种并罚。看完了日本和美国的垃圾分类，是不是觉得我国的垃圾分类还算是比较简单的呢？

Read more from
China Daily, 2020

Read more 2-1

More News Reports for Extensive Learning

What is your rubbish?

On social media platform Weibo, a collection of posts under the topic "你是什么垃圾", which can be translated into both "what's your rubbish" and "what kind of rubbish are you," have generated nearly 20 million views as of today（July 5）.

Read more from
China Daily, 2020

Read more 2-2

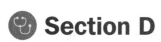

Section D

Projects in Practice【实践探索　行动项目】

1. Project 1

Situational Interaction

Watch the following video（Video 2-2）and discuss within your group how to practice trash sorting as clear as possible.

Video 2-2

2. Project 2

Situational Play:Video-based Practice

(1) Waste separation done right.（Video 2-3）

(2) Waste sorting in Shanghai.（Video 2-4）

(3) Trash sorting at NYU Shanghai.（Video 2-5）

Video 2-3

Video 2-4

Video 2-5

Section E

Self-asessment【进阶评估 自我超越】

1. Cooperative Learning Assessment

Please check your contribution to the group after the project is done.

	Superior (5)	Above Average (4)	Average (3)	Below Average (2)	Weak (1)
Understood what was required for the project					
Participated in the group discussion					
Helped the group to function well as a team					
Contributed useful ideas					
How much work was done					
Quality of completed work					
What could you improve upon next time?					
Your group members' comments					
Your group leader's comments					

2. Assessment of Your Study

Instructions:

(1) Read each statement in the table below and place a check mark in the column that best describes how well you can complete that task.

(2) Review your responses for each task. If you have checked five or more in the "Somewhat" and / or "No" columns, you may need to consider making greater efforts after class.

I can	Yes	Somewhat	No
Understand the main idea of the text			
Identify the major points, important facts and details, and vocabulary in the text			
Make inferences about what is implied in the text			
Recognize the organization and purpose of the text			
Remember the new words and expressions			
Speak on the topic effectively			
Employ search strategy to gain information to address the project			
Refer to appropriate resources to deal with the project			

3. Say What You Want to Say

Please start what you want to say.（Resource 2-3）

Resource 2-3

Unit 2　Household Maintenance

家居保养

Section A

Warm-up Activity【家政服务　赶超潮流】

1. **Read the Following Fashion Brand**

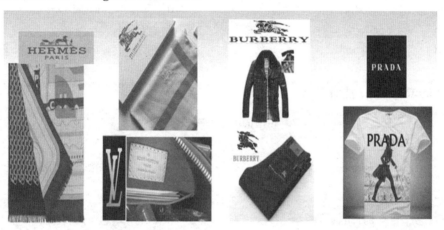

2. **Read the Following Washing Icon**

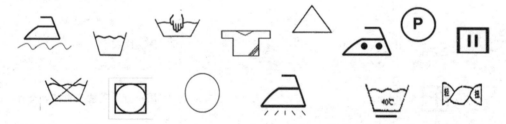

3. **Read More from Fashion Brands**

Understand what the fashion brands are made of.（Video 2-6）

Video 2-6

Section B

Ⅰ Laundry Tips【温馨贴士　关注健康】

1. Cloth Fabric / 衣物材质

材质标识	Cloth Fabric	衣物材质	材质标识	Cloth abric	衣物材质
C	cotton	棉质	L	linen	亚麻
W	wool	羊毛	Ram	ramie	苎麻
WS	cashmere	羊绒	Hem	hemp	大麻
RH	rabbit hair	兔毛	T	polyester	涤纶
S	silk	真丝	MD	modal	莫代尔
MS	mulberry silk	桑蚕丝	LY	lycra	莱卡
Tel	tencel	天丝	N	nylon	锦纶

2. Laundry Tag / 洗涤图标

Instructions / 图标说明		
	washing	水洗:用洗涤槽表示机洗和手洗
	bleaching	漂白:用等边三角形表示
	ironing	熨烫:用熨斗表示
	dry-cleaning	干洗:用圆圈表示
	drying	晾干:用正方形或悬挂的衣服表示
	number stands for the highest temperature	在图案中加数字表示该图形所示动作最高温度
	line stands for the mild process	在图下方加一短线表示该图形所示动作须缓和,加两条线表示必须非常缓和
×	not allowed	图形上加×表示禁止该图形所示动作

	Washing / 水洗	
	washing	水洗
	do not wash	不可水洗
	hand wash	手洗（若未注明洗涤温度，则最高水温不超过90℃）
40℃	washing at max 40℃ mild process	机洗最高水温不超过40℃，中速洗涤
	wash with cold water	冷水机洗
	wash with warm water	温水机洗
	wash with hot water	热水机洗
	Dry-cleaning / 干洗	
	dry-clean	可以干洗
	do not dry-clean	不可干洗
P	any dry-cleaning methods	可用各种干洗剂干洗
A	all usual solvents allowed	适合所有干洗溶剂洗涤
F	dry-clean with petroleum ect.	使用轻质汽油等溶剂干洗

Ironing and Pressing / 熨烫

	iron on low heat at max 110℃	低温熨烫
	iron on medium heat at max 150℃	中温熨烫
	iron on high heat at max 200℃	高温熨烫
	do not iron	不可熨烫
	iron with a press cloth	垫布熨烫
	steam iron only	蒸汽熨烫

Natural Drying / 晾干

	line drying	悬挂晾干
	flat drying	平摊晾干
	drip line drying in the shade	阴干
	drip line drying	悬挂滴干
	twistable	可拧干的
	do not twist	不可拧干

	Bleaching / 漂白	
	bleach	可漂白
	do not bleach	不可漂白
C1	chlorine bleach	可以氯漂
	oxygen / non-chlorine bleach	允许氧漂 / 非氯漂
	Tumble Drying / 烘干	
	tumble drying	可转笼烘干
	do not tumble dry	不可转笼干燥
	tumble drying with low heat, at max 60℃	低温转笼干燥,最高温度不超过60℃
	tumble drying with medium heat, at max 70℃	中温转笼干燥,最高温度不超过70℃
	tumble drying with high heat, at max 90℃	高温转笼干燥,最高温度不超过90℃

3. Household Keeping / 内务整理

Basic Bedding / 寝具必备

用品图标	Name / 名称	用品图标	Name / 名称
	mattress pad 软床垫		comforter 被芯
	mattress topper 床垫罩		blanket 毯子
	pillow 枕头		sheet 床单

Golden Rules of Items to Hang or Fold / 衣物储藏法则

Items to Hang	悬挂衣物
linen, rayon or all-cotton blouses	亚麻、人造丝或全棉的女式衬衫
slippery silks and satins	光滑的绸缎
raw silk, velvet, chiffon, and taffeta	生丝、天鹅绒、雪纺、塔夫绸衣服
suit jackets and blazers	西装夹克,运动外衣
pants with creases	有熨烫折痕的裤子
other dress pants	西装裤
pleated skirts and pants	百褶裙、裤
most dresses	连衣裙
skirts	半身裙
outdoor jackets and overcoats	户外夹克、大衣
bathrobs	浴袍
ties	领带
dressy camisoles and light tank top	紧身背心
Items to Fold	**折叠物品**
knitwear (sweaters of all varieties, plus other knitted pants, skirts and dresses)	针织品(各种毛衣,加上其他针织上衣、裤子、裙子)
bias-cut and A-line skirts and dresses	斜裁的和A字的裙子
cotton T-shirts / Pressed shirts	棉质T恤 / 汗衫
jeans, khakis and corduroys	牛仔裤、卡其布、灯芯绒
scarves and shawls	围巾、披肩
underwear and socks	内衣、袜子
workout clothes and other sportswear	锻炼服和其他运动服

Items for the Guest Room / 客房必备

Items for the Guest Room	客房必备
a list of helpful details about your home	家庭常用清单
a carafe or bottle of water and water glass	准备一瓶水和水杯
interesting fiction and nonfiction books	准备一本有趣的小说和其他类书籍
bedside fan and flashlight	准备床边风扇和手电筒
pad, pensil, and pens	笔和便签条
blow-dryer	吹风机
favorite soaps, shampoos, hand creams, and lotions	客人喜欢的一套清洁护肤用品
Rooms should be personal, attentive, and full of hospitable amenities.	客房应该布置成个人特色的、细心的、好客的。
have plenty of extra bedding	备用的全新床品
If the floors are wood or stone, place a small rug beside the bed.	如果房间地面是木质或石质的，应该在床边放置一小块地毯。
If there is not an adjacent private bathroom, leave a set of towels in the guest room.	如果客房没带浴室，留下一套毛巾在客房。
If the room has closet space, ensure that it is equipped with hangers and a full-length mirror.	如果客房带衣帽间，确保配有足够的衣架挂钩和全身镜。
Include a wastebasket and make sure it is empty before the guest arrives and soon after he / she departs.	准备好一个废纸桶，在客人来之前和出门后清理干净。

Items for Living Room / 客厅备用

Items for Living Room	客厅备用品
newspaper / magazine	报纸 / 杂志
black tea / green tea	红茶 / 绿茶
ice cube / ice tongs	冰块 / 冰夹
tea cup / glass	茶杯
saucer	咖啡碟
napkin paper holder	口纸杯
coaster	杯垫
toothpick	牙签
coatbrush	衣刷
shoe horn	鞋拔
scissors	剪刀
tissue paper	面巾纸
plant	植物盆景
black coffee / white coffee	清咖 / 奶咖
sugar	方糖
water boiler	水壶
rubbish bin	垃圾桶

Items for Bedroom / 卧室备用

Items for Bedroom	卧室备用品
matress	床垫
bed sheet	床单
bed pad	床帕
pillow case	枕头套
duvet	被子
pillow down feather	羽绒枕头
synthetic pillow	合成枕头
duvet cover	被套
blanket	毯子
standing light	落地灯
bed board	床板
suit hanger	西装架
cushion	靠垫
curtain	窗帘
desk lamp	台灯
hanger / skirt hanger	衣架 / 裙架
mat	脚垫

Items for Bathroom / 浴室备用

Items for Bathroom	浴室备用品
bath foam	沐浴露
shampoo	洗发水
bath soap / hand soap	大香皂 / 小香皂
soap dish	肥皂碟
bathtowel / handtowel / facetowel	浴巾 / 中巾 / 小方巾
bathrobe / shower cap / yukata	浴袍 / 浴帽 / 浴衣
bath mat	地巾
hair dryer	吹风机
weight scale	体重秤
toothbrush	牙具
comb / mirror	梳子 / 镜子
shaving kit	须刨
body lotion	润肤露
cotton buds	棉签
emery board	指甲锉
sanitary bag	卫生袋
toilet paper	卷纸

Ⅱ Notes【说文解字　名词注释】

1. Vocabulary Table

Vocabulary 2-2

Words & Expressions	Part of Speech	Meaning in Text
silk	*n.*	真丝
linen	*n.*	亚麻
leather	*n.*	皮质
wool	*n.*	羊毛
cotton	*n.*	棉质
lycra	*n.*	莱卡
modal	*n.*	莫代尔
tencel	*n.*	天丝
iron with a press cloth	*phr.*	垫布熨烫
wash	*vt.*	水洗
hand wash	*phr.*	手洗
drip line drying in the shade	*phr.*	阴干
bleach	*vt.*	漂白
any dry-cleaning methods	*phr.*	可用各种干洗剂干洗
drip line drying	*phr.*	悬挂滴干
do not wash	*phr.*	不可水洗
tumble drying	*phr.*	可转笼烘干
dry-clean	*vt.*	干洗
steam iron only	*phr.*	蒸汽熨烫
washing at max 40℃ mild process	*phr.*	水温不超过40℃，中速洗涤
twistable	*adj.*	可拧干的
iron on medium heat at max 150℃	*phr.*	中温熨烫，不超过150℃
pillow	*n.*	枕头
blanket	*n.*	毯子
sheet	*n.*	床单
knitwear	*n.*	针织品
scarves and shawls	*phr.*	围巾和披肩
underwear and socks	*phr.*	内衣和袜子
bedside fan and flashlight	*phr.*	床边风扇和手电
pad, pensil, and pens	*phr.*	笔和便签条
blow-dryer	*n.*	吹风机
hand creams and lotions	*phr.*	护肤用品
be equipped with	*phr.*	配备
make sure	*phr.*	确保
toothpick	*n.*	牙签
scissors	*n.*	剪刀
tissue paper	*phr.*	面巾纸
sugar	*n.*	方糖

Words & Expressions	Part of Speech	Meaning in Text
rubbish bin	*phr.*	垃圾桶
bed sheet	*phr.*	床单
duvet	*n.*	被子
curtain	*n.*	窗帘
shampoo	*n.*	洗发水
bath soap / hand soap	*phr.*	大香皂 / 小香皂
hairdryer	*n.*	吹风机
weight scale	*phr.*	体重秤
comb / mirror	*n.*	梳子 / 镜子
cotton buds	*phr.*	棉签
sanitary bag	*phr.*	清洁袋
toilet paper	*phr.*	卷纸

2. Useful Knowledge

Laundry Instruction / 洗涤注意事项

Instructions	注意事项
remove stains before washing	水洗前去除污渍
wash separately with different color	颜色不同制品分开水洗
wash with like color	相似颜色制品一同水洗
wash once before wearing	使用前水洗
wash inside out	反面水洗
wet wipe only	仅潮湿擦拭
use the washing bag	使用水洗网
do not soak long time	不可长时间浸泡
dry away from heat	干燥时远离直接热源
shape damp	潮湿时整形
reshape and dry flat	整形后平摊干燥
take it out from the machine as soon as possible after drying	干燥后尽快(从设备中)取出
do not use fluorescent brightener	不可使用荧光增白剂
do not use fabric regulator	不可添加织物调节剂
iron reverse side only	仅反面熨烫
do not iron the ornament	不可熨烫装饰物

Instruction for Different Fabric / 不同材质洗涤注意事项

常见材质	Instructions	注意事项
cotton 棉类	High temperature resistance, separated from colored clothes, hanging in the shade or anti drying.	杜绝高温,与有颜色衣物分开洗涤,阴干。
wool 羊毛类	High temperature washing will shrink, easily yellow and tangled; dry cleaning is the best way; flat drying.	高温下易缩水,易变黄,打结;宜干洗平摊晾干。
silk 丝质类	Hand-wash in cold water, line drying in the shade, using professional detergent.	手洗最佳,阴干,需专用洗涤用品。
linen 亚麻类	Washed by hand, not allowed to wring, ironed at a low temperature.	手洗,不可拧干,低温熨烫。
polyester, nylon, lycra 涤纶,锦纶莱卡	Wash with warm water, iron at low temperature, easy to play electric.	常温水洗,低温熨烫,易带静电。
modal 莫代尔	Soap several minutes before hand wash, gentle mode, do not twist, hang in the shade.	宜手洗,水洗前少时浸泡,轻洗,不可拧绞干,阴干。

3. Idiomatic Usage

(1) remove stains：去除污渍。

(2) wash separately：分开水洗。

(3) wash inside out：反面水洗。

(4) iron reverse side only：仅反面熨烫。

(5) as soon as possible：尽快。

(6) separated from：分开。

(7) high temperature resistance：拒绝高温。

(8) wash with warm water, iron at low temperature, easy to play electric：常温水洗,低温熨烫,易带静电。

4. Background Information

(1) Decoding the care label-how to read the clothing care symbols.（Video 2-7）

(2) Fabric care symbols.（Video 2-8）

Video 2-7

Video 2-8

Section C

Ⅰ Enhanced Learning【深度学习　挑战自我】

1. Matching Game

(　　)(1) Polyester　　　　a. 手洗,不可拧干,低温熨烫。

(　　)(2) Silk　　　　　　b. 宜手洗轻洗不可拧绞干,阴干。

(　　)(3) Wool　　　　　　c. 常温水洗,低温熨烫,易带静电。

(　　)(4) Linen　　　　　 d. 手洗最佳,阴干,需专用洗涤用品。

(　　)(5) Cotton　　　　　e. 杜绝高温,与颜色衣物分开洗涤,阴干。

(　　)(6) Modal　　　　　 f. 高温下易缩水,宜干洗平摊晾干。

Key 2-2

2. Video Learning

Cleaning supplies-list of house cleaning and laundry vocabulary words with pictures in English.（Video 2-9）

Video 2-9

Ⅱ Extensive Learning【拓展学习　媒体动态】

Chanel ends use of exotic skins in its fashion range.

香奈儿宣布旗下时尚产品不再使用鳄鱼皮等珍稀动物毛皮。

Chanel has become the first luxury fashion house in the world to stop using exotic animal skins, like snake, crocodile, lizard and stingray.

香奈儿成为世界首个停止使用蛇、鳄鱼、蜥蜴、魔鬼鱼等珍稀动物皮的奢侈时尚品牌。

Read more from

China Daily, 2020

Read more 2-3

Let's reveal the stories behind.

让我们一起来揭开一些品牌背后的故事。

每个品牌的背后都会有一段故事,是什么让它的logo有了如今的模样,让我们一起来揭开这些品牌背后的故事。

Read more from

TRAMS诠识外语公众号

Read more 2-4

Section D

Projects in Practice【实践探索　行动项目】

1. Project 1

Situational Interaction

Discuss within your group how to practice "Laundry List" as clear as possible.

Laundry List 洗涤工作单

TO / 至: Mary（housekeeper, 家政服务员）

FROM / 由: Mr. Smith（host, 主人）

SUBJECT / 主题: Laundry 洗衣服务

DATE / 日期:_____月 / 日

Message / 正文:

Please do the laundry, following what I ticked out in the laundry list.

Thanks !

(请参照洗衣单上所 ✓ 的项提供相关服务)

□ Washing（水洗）				
□ Dry-cleaning（干洗）				
□ Bleaching（漂白）			
□ Drying（干燥）			
□ Ironing（熨烫）			

2. Project 2

Situational Play: Video-based Practice

(1) What do washing-laundry symbols mean.（Video 2–10）

(2) How to read clothing care labels.（Video 2–11）

Video 2–10

Video 2–11

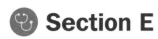 # Section E

Self-assesment【进阶评估　自我超越】

1. Cooperative Learning Assessment

Please check your contribution to the group after the project is done.

	Superior (5)	Above Average (4)	Average (3)	Below Average (2)	Weak (1)
Understood what was required for the project					
Participated in the group discussion					
Helped the group to function well as a team					
Contributed useful ideas					
How much work was done					
Quality of completed work					
What could you improve upon next time?					
Your group members' comments					
Your group leader's comments					

2. Assessment of Your Study

Instructions:

(1) Read each statement in the table below and place a check mark in the column that best describes how well you can complete that task.

(2) Review your responses for each task. If you have checked five or more in the "Somewhat" and / or "No" columns, you may need to consider making greater efforts after class.

I can	Yes	Somewhat	No
Understand the main idea of the text			
Identify the major points, important facts and details, and vocabulary in the text			
Make inferences about what is implied in the text			
Recognize the organization and purpose of the text			
Remember the new words and expressions			
Speak on the topic effectively			
Employ search strategy to gain information to address the project			
Refer to appropriate resources to deal with the project			

3. Say What You Want to Say

Please start what you want to say.(Resource 2-4)

Resource 2-4

Unit 3 Table Etiquette
餐桌礼仪

Section A

Warm-up Activity【餐饮文化　妙趣横生】

1. Read the Following Dining Etiquette

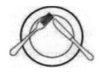

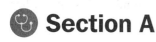

Key 2–3

2. Read Ten Ways How to Fold a Pocket Napkin

Section B

Key 2–4

Ⅰ Table Etiquette【餐桌礼仪　奇思妙解】

1. Ten Pieces from Around the World

In Ireland 爱尔兰

It's considered courteous (礼貌的) to go to the bar to bring back drinks for your entire (整个的) table. Generally, everyone in the group should get up to offer up a round at some point whether you're asked to or not.

In Italy 意大利

In Italy, it's sometimes considered rude to ask for anything that isn't explicitly (明确地) offered to you while dining out, according to Revealed Rome.

In Portugal 葡萄牙

It's OK to add a little extra salt or pepper (胡椒) to your plate as long as the condiments (调味品) are already on the table. But according to a Portugal Travel Guide," asking a server to bring you salt and pepper is considered an offense (冒犯) to the chef's seasoning (调味) skills.

In U.S.A. 美国

In some countries like the U.S.A., it can be considered rude to make sounds when you chew

(咀嚼) or swallow (吞咽) your food. But in Japan, it's a way to show your server or chef that you enjoyed the meal very much.

In France 法国

When in France, splitting the bill with fellow diners should be avoided when possible. You are expected to offer to pay the entire bill or someone else is expected to do so. Of course, according to French Today, there are some instances where splitting the bill is OK, like when dining out with a large group of people or with coworkers (同事).

In Colombia 哥伦比亚

If you're used to cleaning your plate, you might want to consider not doing so when dining in Colombia. It's considered rude to leave an empty plate because it's as if you're telling your host that he or she didn't give you enough food.

In China 中国

In some parts of China, when you reach bone while eating one side of a fish, you must not flip the fish to continue eating. It is said that doing so symbolizes (象征) the capsizing (倾覆) of a fishing boat, according to Culinary Lore. Instead, you should remove the bone and continue eating.

In Australia 澳大利亚

In Australia, people typically prefer not to discuss business matters over a meal. Of course, it depends on the person or group you're with, but you should pay attention to any cues (暗示) from your fellow dining companions (同伴) for good measure.

In Kazakhstan 哈萨克斯坦

In America, it's pretty typical to get annoyed (恼怒的) when your barista (咖啡师) doesn't fill your cup all the up. But in Kazakhstan, it'll actually leave you satisfied since it is a good sign. According to Every Culture, half-filled cups are meant to keep your tea warm since your host will continuously fill your cup as a way to keep the interaction going.

If your host or server were to fill your cup with tea, however, it is a sign that they might want you to leave, according to Commisceo Global.

In Georgian 格鲁吉亚

If you ever find yourself at a supra, which is a traditional Georgian feast, you should avoid sippin (小口喝; 抿) your wine. According to *Georgian Journal*, you should instead wait for the toast and then drink the entire glass

2. Read How to Order Food in English

Key 2-5

Ⅱ Notes【说文解字 名词注释】

1. Vocabulary Table

Vocabulary 2-3

Words & Expressions	Part of Speech	Meaning in Text
Ireland	*n.*	爱尔兰
courteous	*adj.*	礼貌的
entire	*adj.*	整个的
Italy	*n.*	意大利
explicitly	*ad.*	明确地
Portugal	*n.*	葡萄牙
pepper	*n.*	胡椒粉
condiment	*n.*	调味品
offense	*n.*	冒犯
season	*vt.*	调味
chew	*vt.*	咀嚼
swallow	*vt.*	吞咽
coworker	*n.*	同事
Colombia	*n.*	哥伦比亚
symbolize	*vt.*	象征
capsize	*vt.*	倾覆
cues	*n.*	暗示
companion	*n.*	同伴
Kazakhstan	*n.*	哈克萨斯坦
annoyed	*adj.*	恼怒的
barista	*n.*	咖啡师
Georgian	*n.*	格鲁吉亚
sippin	*vt.*	小口喝;抿

2. Useful Knowledge

(1) table etiquette:餐桌礼仪是指人们在赴宴进餐过程中,根据一定的风俗习惯约定俗成的程序和方法,在仪态、餐具使用、菜品食用等方面表现出的自律和敬人的行为,是餐饮活动中需要遵循的行为规范与准则。

(2) 10 pieces of restaurant etiquette from around the world:不同国家有不同的风俗,在餐桌礼仪上更是如此。有些用餐习惯在一个国家可能是文明的,在另一个国家却可能被视作野蛮行为。比如说,在德国,不要用刀切土豆,而应该直接用叉子叉着吃;在日本,不要把筷子插在饭上面;在韩国,不要单手接菜,而要用双手接。世界各国还有哪些值得注意的餐厅礼仪,本文盘点了10个国家的餐厅礼仪。

(3) In Ireland爱尔兰:在酒吧要请同行的人喝一杯。

(4) In Italy意大利:在餐厅主动索要调味品很失礼。

(5) In Portugal葡萄牙:索要盐和辣椒是对厨师的侮辱。

(6) In U.S.A美国:吃饭吧唧嘴是对厨师的尊重。

(7) In France 法国：尽量避免 AA 制。

(8) In Colombia 哥伦比亚：把菜吃光光会让主人面上无光。

(9) In China 中国：给鱼翻面不吉利。

(10) In Australia 澳大利亚：吃饭时不要谈生意。

(11) In Kazakhstan 哈萨克斯坦：倒茶只倒半杯。

(12) In Georgian 格鲁吉亚：在敬酒时一饮而尽。

3. Idiomatic Usage

(1) offer up a round：请同行喝一杯。

(2) splitting the bill：AA 制。

(3) as if：似乎，好像。

(4) flip the fish：给鱼翻身。

(5) keep the interaction going：保持互动。

(6) get annoyed：恼怒，生气。

(7) depend on：依靠，依赖。

4. Background Information

(1) Dishes serving.

Western Dishes Serving / 西餐上菜服务

菜品图标	Serving Order	上菜顺序
	appetizers	开胃菜又称头盘。多用水果、蔬菜、熟肉制成，或用新鲜水产配以美味的沙司和色拉，一般数量较少，常用中小型盘子或冰淇淋杯盛装，色彩鲜艳，装盘美观，令人食欲倍增。开胃菜有冷、热之分，与开胃酒并用。
	soups：consomme or cream	汤有冷汤和热汤之分，也可分为清汤和浓汤，通常法国喜欢清汤，北欧人喜欢浓汤。汤也起开胃的作用，西餐便餐有时选用了开胃品就不再用汤，或者用汤就不选开胃品。
	salads	色拉意为凉拌生菜。色拉可分为水果色拉、素色拉和荤色拉三种。水果色拉常在主菜前上；素色拉大多用醋沙司和色拉油沙司调拌，作为配菜随主菜一起食用；荤色拉多用奶油蛋黄沙司调拌，单独作为一道菜用于宴会冷餐。
	main course	主菜又名主盘，即讲究色、香、味、形。主要原料有鱼贝类、牛、羊、猪肉和禽类。
	dessert：pancake, scone, muffin, pie, tart, butter cake, jelly, ice cream, souffle, pudding	甜食是西餐中的最后一道菜，分软点、干点和湿点三种。软点大都热吃，如煎饼、烤饼、松饼等，作早餐供应为主。干点都是冷吃，如黄油蛋糕、水果馅饼等，一般作为下午茶点。湿点有各种冰淇淋、舒芙蕾、啫喱冻、布丁等，冷热都有，常作午晚餐的点心。
	drinks	饮料一般为咖啡或茶，可加糖和淡奶油。

Chinese Dishes Serving / 中餐上菜服务

菜品图标	Serving Order	上菜顺序
	appetizers: cold dish or mixed food	中餐开胃菜通常是四种冷盘组成的大拼盘。有时种类可多达十种。最具代表性的是凉拌海蜇皮、花生米等。
	soups: shark's fin or chicken soup	一盅浓汤也起开胃的作用,可按实际情况上桌。
	main course	主菜的道数通常是四、六、八等的偶数,因为,中国人认为偶数是吉数。菜肴使用不同的材料,配合酸、甜、苦、辣、咸五味,以炸、蒸、煮、煎、烤、炒等各种烹调法搭配而成。其出菜顺序多以口味清淡和浓腻交互搭配,或干烧、汤类交配列为原则。最后通常以汤作为结束。
	rice / bun	主食通常以大米饭为主,也有由面粉制的馒头和面条作为主食。
	dessert	点心指主菜结束后所供应的甜点,如馅饼、蛋糕、杏仁豆腐等。
	fruits	最后是水果。

Formal Setting / 西餐摆台 (正式)

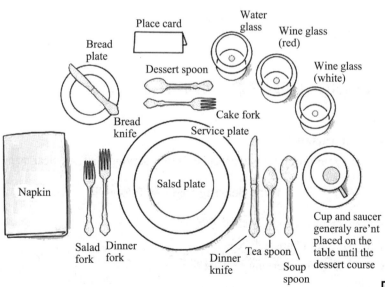

（2）Learn how to set a formal dinner table.（Video 2-12）

Video 2-12

Section C

Ⅰ Enhanced Learning【深度学习　刀叉语言】

Key 2-6

Complete the matching in English.

| Pause | Ready for a Second Plate | Excellent | Do Not Like | Finished |

  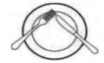 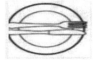

Ⅱ Extensive Learning【拓展学习　媒体动态】

各国餐饮文化差异的思考

I went to a nice restaurant with my parents in Lyon. They were really curious to try something local but they didn't understand a thing on the menu. "Why don't they have pictures?" they asked. In China, lots of menus have photos that illustrate the dishes, so even if you don't understand Chinese, you can still order by pointing at the picture.

我和爸妈去法国里昂的一个高档餐厅吃饭,他们很想尝尝当地特色菜,可是完全看不懂菜单上的菜名。他们问我:"为啥没图片呀?"在中国,很多菜单都附带图片展示菜品的样子,就算你不懂中文,也可以看着图选出你想吃的菜。

Section D

Read more 2-5

Project in Practice【实践探索　行动项目】

1. Project 1

Situational Interaction

Discuss within your group how to practice "Wine Serving List" as clear as possible.

Wine Serving List / 斟酒服务单

TO / 至: Mary（housekeeper, 家政服务员）

FROM / 由: Mr.Smith（host, 主人）

SUBJECT / 主题: Wine Serving 酒单服务

DATE / 日期:＿＿＿＿＿＿＿＿月 / 日

Message / 正文:

Please do some serving, following what I ticked out or crossed in the serving list.

Thanks! (请参照酒单上所√或×的项提供相关服务,谢谢!)

Wine Serving 选酒	☐ Beer / 啤酒	☑ Red Wine / 红酒	☑ Grapes / 葡萄酒	☐ Champagne / 香槟
	☑ Cocktail / 鸡尾酒	☐ Brandy / 白兰地	☐ Soda / 苏打水	☐ Whisky / 威士忌
Wine Serving 温酒	☐ Chilled / 冰镇	☑ Add Ice / 加冰块	☐ Room ℃ / 常温	☑ Chilled / 冰镇
	☐ Chilled / 冰镇	☐ Room ℃ / 常温	☑ Room ℃ / 常温	☐ Chilled / 冰镇

Wine Serving / 斟酒服务

操作	Operating Procedures	操作规范
示酒		站在主人的右侧,左手托瓶底,右手扶瓶颈,酒标朝向主人,让其辨认商标、品种。
温酒		采取升温或降温的方法使酒水的温度适合于饮用。啤酒在4℃—8℃,白葡萄酒在8℃—12℃。
斟酒		斟酒时,瓶口不可搭在酒杯上,相距1厘米为宜。控制好斟酒量,白酒斟八成,红葡萄酒五成,白葡萄酒七成。香槟应分二次斟,第一次斟1/3,待泡沫平息后,再斟2/3处。斟啤酒时,应使酒液顺杯壁滑入杯中呈八成酒二成沫。
续酒		宴食进行中,随时注意添加酒,尤其要注意杯中的酒量,见喝到只剩1/3时,应及时斟满。
饮料		斟有气泡的饮料时,站在客人的右侧沿杯壁徐徐倒入杯中至八成。

2. Project 2

Situational Play:Video-based Practice

(1) 27 napkin fold ideas.（Video 2-13）

(2) Ordering at a restaurant.（Video 2-14）

Video 2-13

Video 2-14

 # Section E

Self-assessment 【进阶评估　自我超越】

1. Cooperative Learning Assessment

Please check your contribution to the group after the project is done.

	Superior (5)	Above Average (4)	Average (3)	Below Average (2)	Weak (1)
Understood what was required for the project					
Participated in the group discussion					
Helped the group to function well as a team					
Contributed useful ideas					
How much work was done					
Quality of completed work					
What could you improve upon next time?					
Your group members' comments					
Your group leader's comments					

2. Assessment of Your Study

Instructions:

（1）Read each statement in the table below and place a check mark in the column that best describes how well you can complete that task.

(2) Review your responses for each task. If you have checked five or more in the "Somewhat" and / or "No" columns, you may need to consider making greater efforts after class.

I can	Yes	Somewhat	No
Understand the main idea of the text			
Identify the major points, important facts and details, and vocabulary in the text			
Make inferences about what is implied in the text			
Recognize the organization and purpose of the text			
Remember the new words and expressions			
Speak on the topic effectively			
Employ search strategy to gain information to address the project			
Refer to appropriate resources to deal with the project			

3. Say What You Want to Say

Please start what you want to say.（Resource 2-5）

Resource 2-5

Unit 4　Home Care

家庭照护

Section A

Warm-up Activity【家庭照护　生命关爱】

1. Read and Practice

Button Menu / 电饭煲按键菜单

Button Menu / 按键菜单	Instructions / 按键说明
start / reheat	启动 / 再加热
cooking timer	定时（预约）
time setting	时间调整
keep warm（select）	保温或保温选择
extended	休眠保温
steam	蒸熟
congee / porridge / soup	稀饭 / 粥 / 汤
white rice	白米饭
sushi	寿司
stewed meat / chicken etc.	炖肉 / 鸡等
brown rice	糙米
fry	烤制
regular	一般煮法
softer	偏软煮法
harder	偏硬煮法
quick cooking	速成煮法
cancel / off	取消；关掉电源

Automatic Electric Cooke / 电饭煲使用

Automatic Electric Cooker / 电饭煲	Instructions / 使用说明
Clean and put the rice into the pan.	把米用其他容器洗净后倒进煲内，不宜用内煲洗米，以免内煲受到碰撞引起变形，影响使用。
Water and marks on the pan： The marks on the left are graduated by the litre. Pour water into the cup up to the mark 0.8 for 0.8 litre of rice. The marks on the right are graduated by the cup. Pour water into up to the mark 4 for 4 cups of rice.	内煲刻度，供放米和水参考刻度用。塑料杯按照1杯米约加1.5杯水的比例。刻度左边以公升为单位，即把量好洗净的米放进煲内，然后加水至该刻度线。例如量米0.8升，水便加到0.8线上。刻度右边以量杯为单位，即如量米4杯，洗净放进煲内加水至4的刻度线。
Place the pan.	放进内煲时，要把内煲左右旋转几次，使它与电热板紧密接触。

Automatic Electric Cooker / 电饭煲	Instructions / 使用说明
No water drop, rice grain, dust are allowed to remain between　bottom and inside of the pan.	内煲底及电热板表面不能附有水滴及饭粒等杂物，以免影响烧饭效果及烧坏元件。
Heat preservation： The temperature of the rice will be kept within 60℃—80℃ after cooking. If preservation is not necessary, pull the plug out of power.	饭煮熟后自动保温在60℃—80℃，如无须保温请拔掉插头。

2. Video Learning

9 surprising facts about eoyal nannies.（Video 2-15）

Video 2-15

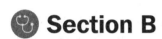 Section B

Ⅰ Parental Care【亲情守护　健康美满】

1. Routines for Child Care

Madrid-born Maria was trained at the prestigious (有声望的) Norland College in Bath, which has educated over 10,000 nannies since it launched (发起) in 1892, for high profile families from Arab royalty to Hollywood stars. Her routines (日常事务) as following.

Bedtime takes place at 7 p.m.

Bedtime takes place at 7 p.m., new foods and flavours (味道) are introduced every few days and playtime takes place outside—come rain or shine. The naughty step is banned and kids are typically in bed at 7 p.m. If the children have travelled on royal engagements (皇室重大活动), it will be difficult getting the kids to bed because of the excitement and the timetable of events.

Not to be a fussy eater

The royal children will not be picky about meals as "you don't have a fussy eater if you have a Norland Nanny" from birth.

Screen time on iPads limited

Screen time on iPads will be limited, and it will be down to the Duke and Duchess of Cambridge as to how long they can play on devices.

No messing

There will be no messing. That's because Maria will be aware that as they step off planes, holding mum's hands, smiling and waving to the crowds, there can't be any crying or tantrums (发脾气). Maria will know their schedule (日程安排). She will be doing a lot of explaining to them, what is happening.

Playtime Schedule

Playtime takes place outside—come rain or shine. Lots of bike rides, playing with their dogs, potentially some gardening.

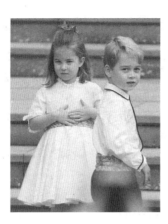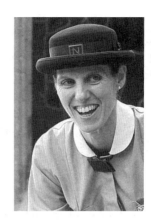

Maria is looking after Princess Charlotte and Prince George.

2. Risk of Skipping Breakfast

Skipping breakfast could raise your risk of heart disease by 87 percent, according to a new study. Researchers at the University of Iowa analyze (分析) 18 years of data on 6,550 people over 40 who had no history of heart disease. They were given regular surveys, which included the question: 'how often do you eat breakfast?' Most (59 percent) ate breakfast every day, but 5.1 percent never did, 10.9 percent rarely did, and 25 percent would skip a few days. The team found a clear link between breakfast habits and heart disease risk. Those who didn't eat in the morning were up to 87 percent more likely to develop heart woes.

"Breakfast is believed to be an important meal of the day, whereas there has been an increasing prevalence (流行) of skipping breakfast over the past 50 years in the United States, with as many as 23.8 percent of young people skipping breakfast every day," the authors write. However, studies on the health effects of skipping breakfast are sparse (稀疏的; 稀少的).

To their knowledge, this is the first retrospective study (回顾性研究) to look at breakfast habits and cardiovascular (心血管疾病) mortality (死亡数; 死亡率).

The team pointed to a few factors which could underlie this connection. First, those who don't eat breakfast may be more likely to snack unhealthily. Second, breakfast may help to balance blood sugar (血糖) levels and control blood pressure. The findings, published on the American College of Cardiology, come days after a similar study showed people who skip breakfast and eat a late dinner are less likely to survive a heart attack.

Skipping breakfast has long been believed as a diet trick (减肥妙招) Joanna Lumley says cutting out breakfast has helped her stay slim in older age. Recently, Twitter CEO Jack Dorsey said he never eats breakfast, only dinner—and that he skips all food altogether on Saturdays as part of a routine that he claims is meditative (沉思的; 冥想的).

Many have suggested that Dorsey's diet could be classed as an eating disorder, rather than, as he puts it, "biohacking".

The new study does not, by any means, provide a concrete verdict (判决; 结论) on breakfast. As Borja Ibáñez, MD, points out in an editorial, association is not necessarily causation. Those who didn't eat breakfast were more likely to smoke, scrimp (精打细算; 吝啬) on exercise, and drink alcohol (酒).

Ⅱ Notes【说文解字　名词注释】

1. Vocabulary Table

Vocabulary 2-4

Words & Expressions	Part of Speech	Meaning in Text
prestigious	adj.	有声望的
launch	vt.	发起
routine	n.	日常事务
flavour	n.	味道
royal engagements	phr.	皇室重大活动
tantrum	n.	发脾气
schedule	n.	日程安排
analyze	vt.	分析
prevalence	n.	流行
sparse	adj.	稀少的；稀疏的
retrospective study	phr.	回顾性研究
cardiovascular		心血管疾病
mortality	n.	死亡数；死亡率
blood sugar	phr.	血糖
a diet trick	phr.	减肥妙招
meditative	adj.	沉思的；冥想的
verdict	n.	判决；结论
scrimp	vt.	精打细算；吝啬
alcohol	n.	酒
pomegranate	vt.	石榴
hyacinth	n.	扁豆
pistachio	n.	开心果
luffa	n.	丝瓜

2. Useful Knowledge

(1) Maria：玛利亚·博拉洛毕业于著名的保姆学校诺兰德学院 (Norland College)，是英国王室特地聘请来协助威廉王子夫妇抚养小王子和小公主的。她接受过十分专业的保姆训练，会讲六国语言。

(2) Norland College：自 1892 年建院以来，诺兰德学院培养了超过一万名保姆，这些保姆为诸如阿拉伯王室、好莱坞明星等著名家庭提供服务。

(3) Madrid：西班牙首都马德里。

(4) be banned：被禁止；不允许。

(5) screen time on iPads：玩电子产品时间。

(6) no messing：意译"不哭不闹"或"学王室礼仪和规矩"。

(7) lots of bike rides and some gardening：经常去骑自行车和做些园艺。

(8) screen time on iPads limited：玩电子产品的时间受限制

(9) playtime schedule：户外玩耍计划。

(10) They were given regular surveys, which included the question："how often do you eat breakfast?" "which" 是定语从句连接词,意指前文的 regular surveys 定期调查。

(11) snack unhealthily：吃不健康的零食。

(12) be less likely to survive a heart attack：心脏病发作时幸存下来的可能性要小一些。其中"less"是"little"的比较级,否定指向,也可理解为"隐性否定"。文本中类似的隐性否定还有"rather than",理解为"而不是"。

(13) association is not necessarily causation：有关联不一定是必然的因果关系。

3. Idiomatic Usage

(1) every few days：每隔几天。

(2) naughty step：淘气。

(3) a fussy eater：挑食者。

(4) be in bed：上床睡觉。

(5) as to：有关,关于。

(6) no messing：不哭不闹。

(7) waving to the crowds：向众人挥手致意。

(8) be aware of / that：知道、意识到。

(9) take place：发生,举行,进行。

(10) come rain or shine：不管刮风下雨。

(11) lots of bike rides and some gardening：经常去骑自行车,做些园艺。

(12) skipping breakfast：不吃早餐。

(13) as many as 23.8% young people：多达23.8%的年轻人。

(14) those who didn't eat in the morning...：那些不吃早餐的人……

(15) be more likely to：更有可能。

(16) blood sugar and blood pressure：血糖和血压。

(17) by any means：无论如何。

4. English-Chinese Translation

(1) Maria is looking after Princess Charlotte and Prince George.（Resource 2-6）

(2) Skipping breakfast could raise risk of heart disease by 87%.（Resource 2-6）

🩺 Section C

Resource 2-6

Ⅰ Enhanced Learning【深度学习　一日感悟】

Frist write, and then learn from each other based on the following topic："A Day in the Life of a Housekeeper".

Ⅱ Extensive Learning【拓展学习 媒体动态】

A Bite of Belt and Road

新闻背景:葡萄、石榴、核桃、香菜……这些都是通过"一带一路"进入中国的。

Grape 葡萄

Originating in the Black Sea and the Mediterranean, the grape entered China from Dayuan, during the reign of Emperor Wu of Han. Dayuan was an ancient country in central Asia, which was famous for grapes.

葡萄最早产于黑海和地中海,在汉武帝时期由大宛传入中国。大宛是中亚地区费尔干纳谷地的一座古城,以盛产葡萄闻名。

Pomegranate 石榴

An Afghan man sells pomegranates along a street in Kabul, Afghanistan. The pomegranate originated in the region of modern - day Iran, and has been cultivated since ancient times throughout the Mediterranean region and northern India. The fruit was introduced to China during the Tang Dynasty (A.D. 618—A.D. 907), and was considered an emblem of fertility and numerous progeny.

石榴产自如今伊朗所在的地区,自古就在地中海地区和印度北部地区培育种植,在唐代(公元618年—公元907年)引入中国。石榴被看作多子多孙的象征。

Walnut 核桃

Brought back by Zhang, the walnut is also known as the longevity fruit. It can warm and invigorate the body, and often serves as a key ingredient in Chinese pastries.

核桃由张骞带入中国,也叫长寿果,能够活血益气,是中式糕点的重要原料。

Garlic 蒜

Garlic is native to the region of southern Europe and central Asia. During the Western Han Dynasty, Zhang introduced the species in the onion genus, Allium, to China.

蒜原产南欧和中亚,属洋葱科葱属植物,在西汉时期,由张骞带入中国。

Cucumber 黄瓜

Cucumber is originally from South Asia, on the southern foot of the Qomolangma Mountain. However, in Zhang's time, the cucumber was known as the "Hu melon".

黄瓜原产于南亚,珠穆朗玛峰南面的山脚地带。在张骞所在的时代,黄瓜被称为"胡瓜"。

Hyacinth Bean 扁豆

The hyacinth was originally grown in India, and brought into China between the Han and Jin dynasties.

扁豆原产于印度,在汉代和晋代时期引入中国。

Pistachio 开心果

The pistachio, a member of the cashew family, was brought into China by the Arabs during the Tang Dynasty.

开心果是腰果家族的一员,在唐代经由阿拉伯人引进中国。

Spinach 菠菜

Spinach is thought to have originated in ancient Persia. The earliest available record of the spinach plant was recorded in Chinese, stating it was introduced into China via Nepal.

菠菜据认为发源于古波斯。现存的有关菠菜的最早史料是用汉字记载的,史料称菠菜是经由尼泊尔引进中国的。

Carrot 胡萝卜

Carrots were originally cultivated for its leaves and seeds. The plant was first introduced into the western parts of China, and then Dunhuang of West China's Gansu province. It was then introduced into the central plains during the Yuan Dynasty (A.D.1271—A.D.1368).

人们原先种植胡萝卜是为了获取它的叶子和种子。胡萝卜最早引入中国西部地区,然后传到甘肃省的敦煌地区。后来在元代(公元1271年—公元1368年)又引入中原地区。

Watermelon 西瓜

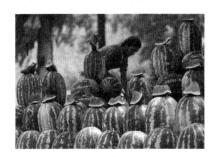

A vendor stands behind watermelons displayed for sale in Kfar Tebnit village, southern Lebanon

Watermelon, which originated in the desert of Africa, was brought along the Silk Road to western China and Ouigour—located in today's Xinjiang Uygur autonomous region—in ancient China. It appeared in Xinjiang during the early Tang Dynasty, and in China's inland between the Five Dynasties, Ten Kingdomgs (A.D. 907—A.D. 960) and Liao Dynasty (A.D. 916—A.D. 1125).

西瓜发源于非洲沙漠地区,经由丝绸之路传到中国西部和古中国的回纥(现新疆维吾尔自治区)。唐朝初期西瓜在新疆出现,五代十国(公元907年—公元960年)和辽代(公元916年—公元1125年)期间传入中国内陆地区。

Luffa 丝瓜

The luffa, which originated in India, was introduced into China during the late Tang Dynasty and became a common vegetable in the Ming Dynasty.

丝瓜发源于印度,唐朝晚期引入中国,明朝时期成为一种常见的蔬菜。

Cabbage 卷心菜

Cabbage, was domesticated in Europe before 1000 B.C. It travelled through the western China before arriving in China by the Hexi Corridor, a part of the Silk Road in Gansu province.

卷心菜是绿色或紫色的二年生叶菜,公元前1000多年开始在欧洲种植。

Don't rush to eat fruit after dinner.
饭后别急着吃水果。

Read more from
TRAMS 诠识外语教学

Read more 2-6

Hese berries can do for you.

Read more from
TRAMS诠识外语教学

Read more 2-7

Section D

Project in Practice【实践探索　行动项目】

1. Project 1
Situational Interaction

Discuss within your group and understand the meaning behind.

双关修辞 (pun) "猜一猜"

(1) An apple a day keeps a doctor away. 传统理解是"一天一苹果,医生远离我",这句话就是用来号召大家多吃苹果的。但这句话还可以用另一种方式来解读:一天一苹果,博士远离我,即"吃苹果会变笨,吃了考不上博士了",因为doctor有两个意思——"医生"和"博士",这种双关让这句话充满喜感。另外,也有人把该句解读为"一天唱一遍《小苹果》,医生也治不了我",这纯粹就是中国式理解了。

(2) Men to the left, because women are always right! 这句话的精妙之处在于 right 这个词。right 有两个意思,一是"对的、正确的",二是"右边的"。比如:You are right. 你是对的。Turn right. 向右转。再回到"Men to the left, because women are always right!",这句话里的 right 兼具"正确的"和"右边的"两种意思,所以这句话可以这样来理解:男人在左边,因为女人总是正确的(言下之意是,女人在右边)。因为这里的 right 具有"双重属性",所以真的很难翻译成中文,大家能不能 get 到里面的梗呢? 当然,美国厕所并不总是"男左女右",波特兰厕所上的这句话也只是一个 joke 而已,不过很妙啊,即指明了男女厕所的方向,又顺带着把女性夸了一番。认识了语言中的"双关"修辞,你就能体会很多英语漫画中的笑点了,也会慢慢爱上英语的。

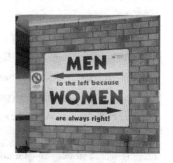

2. Project 2
Situational Play: Video-based Practice
Royal nanny school: the all-round training needed to care for an heir. (Video 2-16)

Video 2-16

Section E

Self-assessment 【进阶评估 自我超越】

1. Cooperative Learning Assessment

Please check your contribution to the group after the project is done.

	Superior (5)	Above Average (4)	Average (3)	Below Average (2)	Weak (1)
Understood what was required for the project					
Participated in the group discussion					
Helped the group to function well as a team					
Contributed useful ideas					
How much work was done					
Quality of completed work					
What could you improve upon next time?					
Your group members' comments					
Your group leader's comments					

2. Assessment of Your Study

Instructions:

(1) Read each statement in the table below and place a check mark in the column that best describes how well you can complete that task.

(2) Review your responses for each task. If you have checked five or more in the "Somewhat" and/or "No" columns, you may need to consider making greater efforts after class.

I can	Yes	Somewhat	No
Understand the main idea of the text			
Identify the major points, important facts and details, and vocabulary in the text			
Make inferences about what is implied in the text			
Recognize the organization and purpose of the text			
Remember the new words and expressions			
Speak on the topic effectively			
Employ search strategy to gain information to address the project			
Refer to appropriate resources to deal with the project			

3. Say What You Want to Say

Please start what you want to say.（Resource 2-7）

Resource 2-7

Chapter 3

A Trip to Lifelong Beauty

生活之"美"

Unit 1 Skin Care
皮肤护理

Section A

Warm-up Activity【掌握"肌"密 守护美丽】

1. True or False: How Much Do You Know About Skin?

(1) The skin is the largest organ in the body.

(2) The outside layer of the skin is dermis.

(3) The size of your pores is determined by the amount of oil they produce.

(4) There are five main skin types: normal, dry, oily, combination and sensitive.

(6) It's important to wear sunscreen even if it's cloudy.

2. Work with a Partner and Analyze Your Partner's Skin Conditions

(1) Use your existing knowledge and experience to analyze your partner's skin conditions.

(2) Use a skincare App to analyze your partner's skin conditions.

(3) Compare the App's analysis results with yours. Let your partner decide which she / he agrees more.

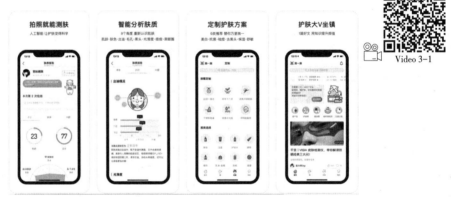

Video 3-1

Section B

Ⅰ Dialogue: Introduction of Facial Care【美容护肤 魅丽一生】

Ms. Wang has made an appointment (预约) for facial (面部护理) treatment at 4:30 p.m. Now the beautician (美容师) at front desk is recommending a facial for her.

A: Beautician No. 1   B: Ms. Wang

A: Hello, madam. How can I help you today?

B: Hello. I'm here for a facial. I made an appointment over the phone for 4:30 today.

A: What's your phone number, madam?

B: 138********.

A: Let me see. Ms. Wang, 4:30, one person.

B: Yes.

A: Which facial would you like, Ms. Wang? We have five different kinds of facials.

B: Which would you recommend?

A: Well, since it's summer and it looks like you've had quite a bit of sun, I'd recommend our summer special (特别项目) —whitening facial.

B: What does it include?

A: This facial starts with deep pore (毛孔) cleansing (清洗) and exfoliating (使皮肤脱皮). Then we'll import whitening serum (精华) to brighten your skin. A LED light therapy (治疗方法) and a whitening mask are followed. We'll finish the facial by applying some of our special cream and sunscreen (防晒霜).

B: That sounds great. How long will the whole facial take?

A: 60 minutes.

B: How much does it cost?

A: 288 yuan per session (一节).

B: OK. I'll have that one then.

A: OK, please follow me.

(Ms. Wang enters the beauty room and begins her facial.)

B: Ms. Wang   C: Beautician No. 2

C: Hello, Ms. Wang. I'm your beautician, Maria.

B: Hello.

C: Please change your clothes and shoes here. The bathrobe (浴袍) and slippers (拖鞋) are all sterilized (对消毒处理).

B: OK.

C: Please take off your jewelry. You can put all your belongings in the locker.

B: OK, thanks.

C: Is the temperature in the room OK?

B: Yes, it's OK.

C: That's good. Please lie down on the bed.

 (Ms. Wang lies down and the facial begins.)

C: First, I'll clean your face with our gentle cleanser (洗面奶). After the cleansing, I'll use the steamer (蒸汽美容仪) to open your pores to bring out the dirt. Then, I'll exfoliate your face to get rid of dead skin cells. After that, I'll import (导入) whitening serum into the skin to lighten your skin and give you a facial massage (推拿) for 20 minutes. I'll use our green LED light to improve your skin tone (色调). At last, I'll apply cream on your whole face to moisturize (润肤) the skin and then some sunscreen to protect it from the sun.

B: OK. I'll have a nap during the treatment.

C: Have a good rest.

(An hour later)

C: The whole facial is done. How are you feeling now?

B: Much better. Thank you.

C: You're welcome. Would you like to get up or continue to lie down and rest?

B: I need to get up. I have work to do.

C: OK. Don't forget your belongings.

B: I won't. Thank you very much.

C: It's my pleasure. See you next time. Have a nice day.

B: You too.

Ⅱ Notes【说文解字　名词注释】

1. Vocabulary Table

Vocabulary 3–1

Words & Expressions	Part of Speech	Meaning in Text
appointment	*n.*	预约
facial	*n.*	面部护理
beautician	*n.*	美容师
special	*n.*	特别项目
exfoliate	*vt.*	使死皮脱落
therapy	*n.*	治疗方法
sunscreen	*n.*	防晒霜
session	*n.*	(某项活动的)一段时间;一场;一节
bathrobe	*n.*	浴袍
slipper	*n.*	拖鞋
sterilize	*vt.*	(美式)对……作灭菌(或消毒)处理
cleanser	*n.*	洗面奶
cleanse	*vt.*	清洗
steamer	*n.*	蒸汽美容仪
pore	*n.*	毛孔
import	*vt.*	导入
serum	*n.*	精华
massage	*n.*	推拿
tone	*n.*	色调
moisturize	*vt.*	(美式)润肤

2. Useful Knowledge

(1) beautician：美容师。美容师是一种专业美容领域的职业称谓,其主要工作在美容院,工作职责是为顾客提供美容服务,比如洗脸、保养、按摩、香薰、和减肥等皮肤护理工作。

(2) front desk：前台,亦可表达为 reception desk。前台的主要工作职责是负责顾客的接待咨询、电话预约、登记服务、档案管理、护理安排、售后回访等。

(3) session：数量单位,表示一次美容护理。course 也是数量单位,表示一个疗程的美容护理。一个疗程的护理由多次护理组成。推销美容项目的时候,一般都是以一个疗程为单位。

(4) open the pores：打开毛孔。虽然用蒸汽打开毛孔是一个常见的美容护理手段,但实际上,用蒸汽"打开"毛孔是一个错误的观念。毛孔的作用就像漏斗,是身体排出多余的油脂和死皮的一个渠道。毛孔没有肌肉,所以也不会像肌肉一样收缩,即不会打开或闭合。蒸汽对毛孔的真正作用在于它分解聚集在毛孔里的"垃圾",如细菌和死皮细胞等,使毛孔清洁更容易。

(5) whiten, brighten, lighten：在美容护肤语境中,这三个词基本表达同一个意思,即美白。在亚洲(尤其是东亚), whiten 广泛使用;但在欧美,由于涉及政治正确和种族多样性和包容性,一般用 brighten 或 lighten 来代替,极少使用 whiten。

(6) skin tone：肤色。

Section C

Ⅰ Enhanced Learning【深度学习　优质服务】

1. 阅读课文,完成填空

(1) You can put all your _____ in the _____.
你可以把自己所有的随身物品放在储物柜里。

(2) Is the _____ OK?
温度还可以吗?

(3) I'll use our green LED light to _____ your _____.
我会用我们的绿色LED灯来改善你的肤色。

(4) I'll _____ on your whole face to _____ the skin.
我会在你的脸上涂面霜,滋润皮肤。

(5) Would you like to _____ or continue to _____ and rest?
你是想起床还是继续躺着休息?

2. 阅读课文,翻译句子

(1) 浴袍和拖鞋都已经消毒。

(2) 首先,我会用温和的洗面奶清洁你的面部。

(3) 我会用美容蒸汽仪打开你的毛孔,排出里面的污物。

(4) 我会帮你去角质,去除死皮。

(5) 我将导入美白精华,使你的皮肤明亮。

Key 3-1

3. 阅读博文,掌握动态

SOKO Glam's Original 10-Step Korean Skincare Routine

The 10-Step is more than a routine—it's a lifestyle that has become a global phenomenon, grounded in ROK's cultural obsession with healthy skin and backed by decades of scientific advancement. It's not about having more products than you can count, but rather about having the right products that do the right things, and using them in the right order.

Step 1　Makeup Remover & Oil Cleanser

Oil cleansers are the base of the Korean skin care routine and the first step of the double cleanse. They're not only relaxing to use; as you gently massage these cleansers in, they also remove makeup and draw out other oil-based impurities, such as sebum, SPF, and pollution.

WHAT IT DOES	HOW TO
Breaks down oil-based debris such as makeup and sunscreen.	Morning and night, gently massage into dry skin, add lukewarm water to emulsify, then rinse.

Step 2　Water Based Cleanser

The second step of the double cleanse. Cleansing twice is recommended by aestheticians and dermatologists because it helps to thoroughly remove any impurities that can cause breakouts. Water-based cleansers dissolve the water-based impurities such as dirt and sweat that your oil cleanser didn't pick up.

WHAT IT DOES	HOW TO
Removes water-based impurities such as sweat and dirt.	Morning and night, apply to your damp face and neck and massage in a circular motion, then rinse with lukewarm water.

Step 3　Exfoliator

Physical and chemical exfoliation help clean pores and slough off dead skin cells for visibly brighter and smoother skin. Regular exfoliation will also help your other skin care products absorb and work more efficiently!

WHAT IT DOES	HOW TO
Cleans debris from pores and removes dead skin cells.	Gently exfoliate 1–2 times / week, focusing on your nose and the visible pores on your cheeks.

Step 4　Toner

Toners are the ultimate prep product, removing any leftover residue from your cleansers while also repairing your skin's barrier to effectively absorb the moisturizers that follow.

WHAT IT DOES	HOW TO
Balances moisture and pH levels.	Use a cotton pad to swipe all across your face or pat gently into your skin using your hands.

Step 5　Essence

Essences are lightweight and packed with a concentrated blend of hydrating, anti-aging, and complexion-enhancing ingredients

WHAT IT DOES	HOW TO
Hydrates and aids in cell turnover.	Sprinkle into hands and lightly pat into face and neck.

Step 6　Treatments

Boosters, serums, and ampoules are the ultimate skin perfectors. Packed with powerhouse ingredients, they target specific skin concerns such as acne, fine lines, and hyperpigmentation.

WHAT IT DOES	HOW TO
Directly treats problem area.	Gently tap into skin, focusing on areas affected by skin concern.

Step 7　Sheet Mask

Sheet masks are the soul of the Korean skincare routine. The key to sheet masks is the sheet, which when in prolonged contact with your face allows the skin to fully absorb the nutrients and moisture.

WHAT IT DOES	HOW TO
Infuses your skin with concentrated essence.	Smooth onto clean skin, lie back and relax for 15-20 minutes, then pat in excess essence.

Step 8　Eye Cream

The skin around your eyes is the thinnest and most delicate on your face, and regularly using an intensive eye cream can keep dark circles, puffiness, and crow's-feet at bay. Eye creams are concentrated with beneficial ingredients and formulated to be extra gentle and non-irritating.

WHAT IT DOES	HOW TO
Hydrates and prevents dark circles, puffiness, and crow's feet.	Use your pinkie to gentle tap (never rub!) around the entire orbital bone, avoiding the water line.

Step 9　Moisturizer

They come in many forms (emulsion, lotion, gel, cream, and sleeping mask) and seal in moisture to plump up skin and smooth fine lines.

WHAT IT DOES	HOW TO
Seals in moisture to plump and smooth skin.	Pat into your face and neck morning and night, every day.

Step 10　Sunscreen

You should always wear sunscreen, even if you'll be inside most of the day. It's the easiest and most effective way to prevent premature aging (and skin cancer!). Sunscreen should be your last step so it can shield your skin without being diluted by additional products.

WHAT IT DOES	HOW TO
Protects the skin from damaging UV rays.	Gently pat into your face and neck as the last step in your morning routine. Re-apply throughout the day.

Video 3-2

(*Source:* https://sokoglam.com/)

Ⅱ　Extensive Learning【拓展学习　媒体动态】

The seemingly odd coupling of men and makeup is quietly changing the definition of masculinity.

If you consider buying a gift for your father or better half, why not add facial masks or anti-aging cream to your gift list on top of razors and smart gadgets?

It turns out that the skin care market for men in China has enjoyed over 50 percent growth for two consecutive years from 2016 to 2018, according to Alibaba's Tmall platform.

Notably, last year, sales of cosmetics for men surged 89 percent year-on-year on Tmall, higher than that of facial lotions, fragrances and oral hygiene products, though those items also experienced tremendous growth, the company said in an annual report on beauty trends.

Read more from
China Daily, 2019

Read more 3-1

Chinese women are splashing out more on beauty products, and at an earlier age than ever. As increasingly sophisticated consumers, they are pushing an already enormous global industry to new heights and reinforcing the rise of Asian-born companies in the sector.

According to a recent survey by OC&C Strategy Consultants, 88 percent of respondents increased their skincare spending in the last year. The study also found that 90 percent of respondents aged 18 to 24 started using skin-care products before the age of 20.

In China in 2016 retail sales of skin-care products were worth 169 billion yuan ($26.8 billion) and retail sales of makeup products were worth 28.3 billion yuan.

Even with these numbers and very quick growth, China's skin-care spending per capita is still very low compared with other major markets.

Read more from
China Daily, 2018

Read more 3-2

Section D

Projects in Practice【实践探索　行动项目】

1. Project 1

Ad. Reading Comprehension: 美容项目表阅读

The beauty salon, in Beauty Studio, is having a promotion campaign. It's offering a 20% discount for all the services and products. You're a beautician from inBeauty Studio. Please read the ad. below and answer the following questions.

(1) If your customer wants to do one session of eye treatment, how much does she/ he need to pay?

(2) If your customer wants to do one course of deep cleansing facial, how much does she/ he need to pay?

(3) If a teenager with oily skin wants to experience a skin treatment, which one would you recommend? And why?

(4) If your customer is a college freshman and just finish military training, which skin treatment (s) would you recommend?

(5) What can your customer enjoy during the whitening facial treatment?

(6) For customers aged 40 and above, which skin treatment would you recommend?

(7) What can customers expect from an Acne Facial? How many visits do customers need to see the results?

(8) If your customer is hesitant to spend thousands on skin care at a time, what would you say to convince her / him to make the investment?

FACIAL TREATMENT		
Would you like to have a facial treatment? Come to inBeauty Studio for beauty treatment and relaxation. For sure you will feel good. Now we are having 20% off!		
Items	**What Included**	**Pricing**
Eye Treatment	• Massage eye areas to relax eye muscles, reduce wrinkles and dark circles. • Use machine to lift the skin around the eyes. • Apply a cooling mask.	• One session (30 mins)/ ￥250.
Deep Cleansing Facial	• Cleanse skin thoroughly. • Steam face to "open" pores. • Exfoliate dead skin cells. • Extract clogged pores, blackheads, and whiteheads. • Apply a hydrating mask and moisturize skin.	• One session (60 mins)/ ￥360. • One course (a series of 10 sessions) /￥3,200.
Relaxing Facial	• Deep cleansing with aromatic cream. • Exfoliate and cleanse the skin. • Pressure point massage on face, neck and shoulders.	• One session (60 mins)/ ￥360 • One course (a series of 10 sessions)/ ￥3,200.
Whitening Facial	• Exfoliate dead skin cells. • Import whitening serum into the skin to lighten and improve skin tone. • Have LED light therapy. • Apply whitening mask to brighten the skin.	• One session (90 mins)/ ￥400 • One course (a series of 10 sessions)/ ￥3,600.
Collagen Facial	• Cleanse and exfoliate skin. • Massage skin with a collagen cream. • Use machine and lifting cream to tighten and lift the skin's surface to reduce signs of aging. • Apply pure collagen mask.	• One session (90 mins)/ ￥480. • One course (a series of 10 sessions)/ ￥4,500.
Acne Facial	• Thoroughly cleanse face and exfoliate dead skin cells. • Extract blackheads, dirt and oil from clogged pores. • Massage face to calm the skin. • Apply a mask to treat acne. • Apply moisturizer appropriate for acne.	• One session (90 mins)/ ￥480. • One course (a series of 10 sessions)/ ￥4,500.

2. Project 2
Role Play: 角色扮演

Ms. Wang is at a cosmetics counter in a department store. She asks a beauty assistant for a recommendation about skincare products.

A: Beauty Assistant   B: Ms. Wang

A: Hello. How can I help you today?

B: I have a problem with my skin. I'm not sure if I have oily skin or dry skin. Some parts of my face always seem greasy, while others are extremely dry.

A: It sounds like you have combination skin. Let me have a closer look at your skin.

B: OK.

A: Your T-zone is oily, especially your nose. And the pores on your nose are a bit large.

B: Yes, they are always getting clogged. I often break out in acne, too.

A: Your cheeks are quite dry. You do have combination skin. Typically, this type of skin is the hardest to take care of.

B: What should I do?

A: It's very important to keep your skin hydrated all the time. It's better to use moisturizing cream twice a day.

B: Can you recommend some effective creams?

A: I suggest this facial moisturizer. It deeply nourishes your skin. Besides, it improves the pores on your skin. Your skin will appear softer, smoother and younger.

B: Great. Thanks.

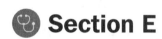 Section E

Self-assessment【进阶评估　自我超越】

1. Cooperative Learning Assessment

Please check your contribution to the group after the project is done.

	Superior (5)	Above Average (4)	Average (3)	Below Average (2)	Weak (1)
Understood what was required for the project					
Participated in the group discussion					
Helped the group to function well as a team					
Contributed useful ideas					
How much work was done					
Quality of completed work					
What could you improve upon next time?					
Your group members' comments					
Your group leader's comments					

2. Assessment of Your Study

Instructions:

(1) Read each statement in the table below and place a check mark in the column that best describes how well you can complete that task.

(2) Review your responses for each task. If you have checked five or more in the "Somewhat" and / or "No" columns, you may need to consider making greater efforts after class.

I can	Yes	Somewhat	No
Understand the main idea of the text			
Identify the major points, important facts and details, and vocabulary in the text			
Make inferences about what is implied in the text			
Recognize the organization and purpose of the text			
Remember the new words and expressions			
Speak on the topic effectively			
Employ search strategy to gain information to address the project			
Refer to appropriate resources to deal with the project			

3. Personal Development

Instruction:

Completing this section will help you make informed practicing decisions. Please identify your strengths and the areas that you need to develop or strengthen and record them below.

STRENGTHS: I am confident that I can...
(1)
(2)
(3)
AREAS FOR IMPROVEMENT: I would like to improve my ability to...
(1)
(2)
(3)

4. Say What You Want to Say

(1) What's your skin type? What's your skin care routine?

(2) What do you think are the most important qualities of a beautician?

Unit 2　Body Care
美体保健

Section A

Warm-up Activity【专业专注　匠心守护】

1. Look at the Pictures and Match Them with the Right Words

massage bed　　　pillow　　　towels　　　essential oil　　　blanket

    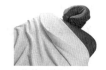

2. Listen to Robert Trying to Convince Staci to Have a Message and Answer the Following Questions

(1) Why do Staci's back and shoulders hurt?

(2) What does Staci dislike about massage?

(3) If the massage therapists are too rough, what can Staci do?

(4) Why does Robert recommend his massage therapist?

(5) When do you think will Staci really go to get a massage?

Video 3–3

Section B

Ⅰ Dialogue: Body Care Service Process【舒体舒心　健康无忧】

(Mr. Zhang is twisting his back all the time. Therefore, he goes to a beauty salon for help.)

A: Beautician　B: Mr. Zhang

A: What can I do for you, Mr. Zhang?

B: My neck is stiff (僵硬的). I feel aches in my back and shoulders.

A: I see. You need a good massage. It will get rid of the knots (结节) in your muscles and relieve your pain.

B: Good. How long will it take?

A: The massage will last one hour.

B: How much does it cost?

A: 168 yuan.

B: OK. I'll have one.

A: Please change your outfits first. Here are sterilized pajamas and slippers. I will go make preparations (准备工作) and come back in five minutes.

B: Alright.

(Five minutes later, the beautician knocks the door.)

A: Mr. Zhang, may I come in?

B: Yes, come on in please.

A: Please take off the pajama top and lie face down. Is the temperature OK?

B: Yes. It's good.

(The massage begins with long, smooth (流畅的) and gentle strokes (抚摸))

A: First I'm warming your tissue (组织). Then I'll massage essential oil (精油) into your skin and work more deeply.

B: Essential oil?

A: Yes. A few drops of essential oil can be really helpful. They can help loosen (使松弛) up your muscles and alleviate (减轻) your pain.

B: Oh. That sounds great. Is it smelly? I don't like smelly essential oil.

A: Don't worry. It smells good. If you really don't like the smell, I'll stop using it.

B: Thank you.

A: Now how do you feel?

B: I'm alright.

A: During the massage, I'll check in with you (和······确认) two or three times. If the pressure is not ok, please speak up.

B: OK.

(During the massage)

A: All right, sir. How's the pressure? Do you need me to press harder or softer?

B: I think it's alright.

A: OK. Now the neck area is done. Before I move on, do you feel like I got all the sore (疼痛的) spots? Or is there anything that needs more attention?

B: Would you please pinch (捏) here harder?

A: No problem.

B: I feel much better now.

(An hour later)

A: The massage is over. Now I will use the towel to clean your skin. How do you feel?

B: I feel much relaxed now.

A: That's good. I'll cover you with a blanket (毯子). You can lie back down and have a rest.

B: Thank you.

A: You're welcome.

II Notes【说文解字　名词注释】

1. Vocabulary Table

Vocabulary 3-2

Words & Expressions	Part of Speech	Meaning in Text
stiff	*adj.*	僵硬的
knot	*n.*	结节
preparation	*n.*	准备工作
smooth	*adj.*	流畅的
stroke	*n.*	抚摸
tissue	*n.*	(动植物的)组织
essential oil	*phr.*	精油
loosen	*vt.*	使松弛
alleviate	*vt.*	减轻(痛苦等)
check in with sb.	*phr.*	和……确认
sore	*adj.*	疼痛的
pinch	*vt.*	捏
blanket	*n.*	毯子

2. Useful Knowledge

(1) ache, hurt, pain 均表示疼痛。

(2) lie face down：趴下。与其相对的是 lie back down 躺下。这两个是基本的行为指令。

(3) essential oil：精油。精油是从植物中提炼萃取的挥发性芳香物质。用稀释过的精油进行按摩是美容院的基本操作之一。精油可以刺激血液和淋巴循环,提升免疫系统,舒缓紧张,压力,放松肌肉等。常见的精油有薰衣草精油 (lavender oil),玫瑰精油 (rose oil),甘菊精油 (chamomile oil),薄荷精油 (peppermint oil) 和橄榄油 (olive oil) 等。

(4) relieve, alleviate, ease 均表示缓解,常见搭配 relieve / alleviate / ease pain 缓解疼痛。

(5) pressure：力道。在身体护理过程中,美容师应该询问顾客是否满意按摩力道,从而做出相应调整,避免造成伤害。比较常用且有效的询问方式分三步走。第一步,用一句 all right 来吸引顾客注意:在按摩过程中有些顾客昏昏欲睡,所以需要先让他们回神。第二步,用"How's the pressure?"或"Is the pressure OK?"或"Are you feeling too strong?"把目的传达给顾客——美容师想要了解力道是否合适。但由于不少顾客会不好意思表达自己的真实想法,所以美容师要给顾客提供选择。因此,第三步,用一个选择疑问句:"Do you need me to press harder or softer?"或"Would you like a bit more or less?"或"Do you need increase / decrease the pressure?"

(6) Before I move on, do you feel like I got all the sore spots? Or is there anything that needs more attention? 我将转移到你身体的另一个区域了,我刚刚推拿的位置你还有哪里感到疼痛的吗？或者哪里需要我再推拿一下？在身体护理过程中,美容师和顾客应该保持有效的沟通。在每一个身体部位推拿完前,美容师应该总结性地询问一下顾客是否满意或者哪里需要再加强。

Video 3-4

Section C

I Enhanced Learning【深度学习　修身养性】

1. 护肤产品,选词填空

| massage cupping repair circulation essential |
| pregnant reflexology stress healing |

(1) _____ women should be cautious about massage.

(2) _____ oil is extracted from plants and has healthful effects.

(3) The suction provided by _____ can loosen muscles and encourage blood flow.

(4) Moxibustion can help move stagnant energy in the body and increase the blood _____. Therefore, it can treat menstrual irregularities.

(5) _____ involves pressing different areas on the feet that are connected to specific organs and body parts.

2. 阅读课文,翻译句子

(1) 我的脖子僵硬,肩膀和背部疼痛。

(2) 消除结节。

(3) 精油可以放松肌肉,缓解疼痛。

(4) 如果你对按摩力道不满意,请开口。

(5) 你需要我特别留意什么部位?

Key 3-2

3. 阅读博文,掌握动态

Spa Etiquette in China: Clothing, Tipping, and Services

Getting a spa treatment in China is a wonderful luxury. Unlike in many parts of the world, spas and massage parlors are very common in most neighborhoods of major cities across the country. While there are high-end options, there are also many local shops that provide clean, comfortable, and excellent services for natives and foreigners.

For first-timers, a visit to a spa in China can be a stressful experience as they are unfamiliar with the customs and etiquette. Never fear! Knowing the answers of how to act and what to expect before heading into the spa, will allow you to focus on the important part-relaxing.

Clothing at the Spa

Should you disrobe entirely at a spa? The answer depends on where you are and what you're doing. Most Chinese massages, e.g. foot massage, traditional massage, at small spas or even the local ones, will offer pajamas to put on.

If the spa caters to Westerners, the outfit should be larger and you shouldn't have any trouble. If it's a local place, and you're a big person, then you may want to ensure it will fit before disrobing.

Generally, your therapist will lead you to your therapy room and point out where you are supposed to change and what they would like you to wear. If not, have a good look around the room. Don't be shy and ask questions if you're unsure.

Other types of spas and specific treatments like a full-body oil massage, require nudity. When in doubt, ask. You'll have to be a little immodest and brave, but you can mime to the therapist and ask if you should take everything off. You'll be guided to the robe, paper (disposable) underwear or other garments to wear. Your therapist will discreetly leave the room and knock before entering to give you privacy.

Bathhouse Etiquette

Bathhouses require you to walk around completely nude except for slippers and a locker key. You'll leave your clothing in a locker and then be guided to a shower area to wash away the day's grime. Some bathhouses and hot springs carefully monitor the cleansing part of the routine. Then strut your stuff around to the various soaking pools, steam rooms, and scrub rooms. You will not be alone in your nudity and you'll get used to it fast. For the public areas, visitors are given cotton pajamas to wear.

Many English-language spa websites have lists of rules and frequently-asked questions. To prepare for your spa adventure, go over the information on the websites and plan to arrive early to ask any questions you may have.

Tipping

Tipping in China is different than in the United States. Unlike spas in the West, you are not expected to tip at spas in China. If you have a treatment at an international hotel, there will be a hefty service charge added, but an extra gratuity is not expected.

Booking

Depending on what kind of spa you're visiting, you don't always need to book in advance. If you're in the middle of a shopping trip or walking tour and pass a reflexology spot (there will be a giant image of a foot on a sign outside) you can easily pop in for an hour's foot massage without booking in advance. At hotel spas and popular spots chains, it's better to book in advance.

Video 3-5

Ⅱ Extensive Learning【拓展学习　媒体动态】

Of all the weight-loss techniques out there, the idea that regular massages could help you shed pounds is definitely among the most appealing. It seems too good to be true-all you have to do is lie there and the weight starts to fall off? Well, that's not exactly how it works.

"In my 15 years as a massage therapist, I've helped a lot of people lose some serious weight," says Wil Lewis, massage program director at New York City's Chillhouse. But he's quick to add that massages alone aren't what helped clients lose weight. Rather, his methods set clients up for success by putting them in the proper mental and physical space to effectively diet and exercise.

Weight loss can often be seen as a tough and miserable pursuit that hinges on pain and suffering, says Lewis. But when massage is incorporated into that weight-loss plan, there's suddenly an element of self-love and care. In his experience, Lewis says that massage therapy can make the process of weight loss more positive, which encourages people to stick with it. Plus, a massage is an excellent non-food reward for when you reach your goals.

Read more from
Women's Health, 2017

Read more 3-3

When it comes to getting the most out of your trip to a resort or day spa, booking the right types of massage go a long way in making sure you return from your vacation relaxed, healthy, and in less pain than when you arrived.

Reflexology is an often misunderstood and overlooked spa treatment where the therapist works on reflex points on your feet, hands, and ears that are thought to relate to specific organs and glands in the body. By stimulating these points with finger pressure, massage therapists claim to be able to promote health in those organs and glands via the body's energetic pathways.

When done by a skilled practitioner, reflexology is a deeply relaxing treatment with benefits that can be felt throughout the body. The therapist will use various techniques that include holds, finger pressure, kneading, rotation, and rubbing, so be prepared for a very intimate experience if you book one of these treatments at your spa or resort.

Read more from
Trip Savvy, 2019

Read more 3-4

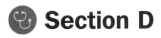 Section D

Projects in Practice【实践探索　行动项目】

1. Project 1

Design A Poster:店庆海报设计

Your beauty salon is having its 10th anniversary celebration and having special offers in order to express gratitude to regular customers and attract new customers. Please design an English poster to promote the celebration.

2. Project 2
Role Play：角色扮演

Work with a partner. Based on the text, adjust the dialogue by changing the customer demand and treatment. Act out the dialogue.

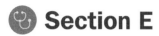 # Section E

Self-assessment【进阶评估　自我超越】

1. Cooperative Learning Assessment

Please check your contribution to the group after the project is done.

	Superior (5)	Above Average (4)	Average (3)	Below Average (2)	Weak (1)
Understood what was required for the project					
Participated in the group discussion					
Helped the group to function well as a team					
Contributed useful ideas					
How much work was done					
Quality of completed work					
What could you improve upon next time?					
Your group members' comments					
Your group leader's comments					

2. Assessment of Your Study
Instructions:

(1) Read each statement in the table below and place a check mark in the column that best describes how well you can complete that task.

(2) Review your responses for each task. If you have checked five or more in the "Somewhat" and / or "No" columns, you may need to consider making greater efforts after class.

I can	Yes	Somewhat	No
Understand the main idea of the text			
Identify the major points, important facts and details, and vocabulary in the text			
Make inferences about what is implied in the text			
Recognize the organization and purpose of the text			
Remember the new words and expressions			
Speak on the topic effectively			
Employ search strategy to gain information to address the project			
Refer to appropriate resources to deal with the project			

3. Personal Development

Instruction:

Completing this section will help you make informed practicing decisions. Please identify your strengths and the areas that you need to develop or strengthen and record them below.

STRENGTHS: I am confident that I can...
(1)
(2)
(3)
AREAS FOR IMPROVEMENT: **I would like to improve my ability to...**
(1)
(2)
(3)

4. Say What You Want to Say

(1) What are the most important qualities of communications between customer and beautician?

(2) If a customer makes some inappropriate moves, how will you as a beautician / manager handle the situation?

Unit 3　Medical Beauty Service

医美服务

Section A

Warm-up Activity【整容时代　我型我塑】

1.　Read the Following Phenomenon and Answer the Questions

Asians, especially the people of ROK and Chinese are obsessed with fair skin, bigger eyes with double eyelids, well-defined nose and V-shaped chin. This kind of look can be achieved by cosmetic surgeries. Therefore, thousands of Asians have turned to the knife or needle to change their looks.

Video 3-6

(1)　Why do you think Asians are obsessed with this specific look?

(2)　What are the advantages and disadvantages of cosmetic surgeries?

2.　Conduct a Mini Survey on Your Knowledge and Attitudes About Cosmetic Surgery

What do you know about these kinds of cosmetic surgery? Would you try them? Complete this table with your partner.

Cosmetic Surgery	What do you know?	Would you try it? Why or Why not?
Double Wyelids		
Facelift		
Nose Job		
Breast Augmentation		
Tummy Tuck		
Hair Transplant		
Liposuction		

Section B

Ⅰ Dialogue: Customer Consultation Service【重塑美丽　提升自信】

(Ms. Yang comes to the plastic surgery clinic and consults an adviser about the double eyelids surgery)

A: Consultant　B: Ms. Yang

A: Good morning, Ms. Yang. How can I help you?

B: Hello. I'd like to have a consultation (咨询) about my double eyelids (眼睑) surgery (外科手术). I want to know everything about the surgery.

A: OK, Ms. Yang. Have you ever had double eyelids surgery before?

B: No. Actually I don't have any plastic surgeries before.

A: All right. How did you happen to choose us for consultation?

B: I heard that the doctors and nurses in your clinic are all qualified (有资格的) professionals (专业人士) with official certifications (证书).

A: Yes. You can put your trust in us. As for double eyelids surgery, it is the most popular surgery in our clinic (诊所). We have done a tremendous (大量的) number of surgeries and the customers are happy about the results.

B: That's good to hear. How many types of surgery are there?

A: There are two major types. One is the full incision (切口) eyelid surgery. It's the most common type. It's famous for producing the most natural look for the long term.

B: It sounds great.

A: Yes, indeed. However, there is a downside (缺点). It takes times for you to heal and get natural.

B: Good things take time. What is the other one?

A: The other type is buried sutured (缝合的) eyelid surgery. It is non-invasive (非侵入的) and non-incision. The surgery time is very short and the swelling (肿胀) disappears in two to three days after surgery.

B: Wow, it's quick.

A: Yes. That's why it's very popular for people who have limited time.

B: What's the downside of this surgery?

A: Well, it's not suitable for heavy fat or muscle eyes.

B: Which one suits me better?

A: It will be decided during face-to-face consultation with your doctor.

B: OK. How long is the operation?

A: From 30 minutes to one hour. After the surgery, you will stay for a couple of hours at the clinic and then you can leave.

B: Will anesthesia (麻醉) be used?

A: Yes. The doctor will discuss the specific details with you.

B: How long is recovery (恢复) after surgery?

A: It varies from person to person. Most of the swelling and bruising (瘀伤) will disappear with two to four weeks after surgery. Overall, double eyelid surgery recovery process (过程) as a whole is relatively slower than other surgeries.

B: When will I begin to look "normal" again?

A: It will take at least three months to look natural in person. The whole process will take six months to one year. Then you will look flawlessly natural.

B: What should I pay attention to before the surgery?

A: You need to stop taking certain medications (药物) one to two weeks before the surgery. Here, on this booklet (小册子), we list all the medications you should avoid. Stop smoking two weeks before the surgery.

B: OK. It's easy to do. How do I perform post-operative (手术后的) care?

A: Apply iced gauze pads (冰纱布垫) to your eyes and cheeks for the first 48 hours. Take only medications prescribed (开处方) by your doctor. Avoid extreme physical activity. You should also avoid wearing makeup within the first ten days. You can find all the pre and post-operative instructions on our booklet.

B: Thank you. I'll read it carefully. How much does the surgery cost?

A: It's around 4000 yuan.

B: It's quite reasonable (合理的). Please make an appointment with the doctor for me as soon as possible.

A: OK. I will do it right now.

B: Thank you. See you next time.

A: You're welcome. Please don't forget the booklet. See you soon.

Video 3-7

Ⅱ Notes【说文解字　名词注释】

1. Vocabulary Table

Vocabulary 3-3

Words & Expressions	Part of Speech	Meaning in Text
consultation	*n.*	咨询；就诊
eyelid	*n.*	眼睑；眼皮
surgery	*n.*	外科手术
qualified	*adj.*	（通过考试）取得资格的；有资格的；合格的
professional	*n.*	专业人士
certification	*n.*	证书
clinic	*n.*	诊所
tremendous	*adj.*	大量的
incision	*n.*	切口
downside	*n.*	负面；阴暗面；缺点
suture	*v.*	缝合伤口

Words & Expressions	Part of Speech	Meaning in Text
non-invasive	*adj.*	非损伤的；非侵入的
swelling	*n.*	肿胀；浮肿
anesthesia	*n.*	麻醉
recovery	*n.*	(身体的)恢复；康复
bruising	*n.*	瘀伤；青肿
process	*n.*	过程
medication	*n.*	药物；药
booklet	*n.*	小册子
post-operative	*adj.*	手术后的
iced gauze pads	*phr.*	冰纱布垫
prescribe	*v.*	开(药、处方)
reasonable	*adj.*	(价钱)合理的；公道的；不太贵的

2. Useful Knowledge

(1) full incision eyelid surgery：双眼皮全切手术。通过切口，去除松弛的皮肤、眼轮匝肌及肥厚的脂肪，在直视下直接将皮肤同眼轮匝肌或提上睑肌腱膜缝合到一起，形成重睑。此方法需切开皮肤，创伤略大，但通过切口可做上睑结构的调整，效果可靠、持久，适合于各种情况下的单睑。缺点是操作较复杂，创伤较大，术后需要一定的时间让水肿消退。

(2) buried sutured eyelid surgery：双眼皮埋线手术。通过缝合方式，直接把缝线埋藏于皮肤及睑板之间，使上睑皮肤同睑板发生粘连，形成重睑。此手术操作简便，创伤小，不留疤痕，消肿快，不需拆线，比较适合年轻人的眼皮较薄、眼裂长、无皮肤松弛的情况；对眼皮较厚，皮肤松弛及年龄较大者不太适合，并有重睑消失的可能。

(3) non-invasive：非侵入性的。非侵入性手术被定义为任何不需要通过切口或穿刺皮肤或通过体腔进入人体的外科手术。双眼皮手术中，埋线手术是非侵入性的，全切手术则是侵入性的。

(4) anesthesia：麻醉。双眼皮手术主要使用局部麻醉 (local anesthesia)，通过镇静注射 (sedation) 的方式。

(5) It varies from person to person. 双眼皮手术恢复期因人而异。手术类型、术后护理的质量以及个人体质都能影响恢复期的长短。

Video 3-8

Section C

Ⅰ Enhanced Learning【深度学习　打造完美】

1. 医美整容,连线搭配

(1) 丰唇　　　　　　　　　　a. laser resurfacing

(2) 双下巴去除术　　　　　　b. Botox injection

(3) 鼻梁鼻头整形　　　　　　c. lip augmentation

(4) 肉毒杆菌注射　　　　　　d. double chin reduction

(5) 激光焕肤　　　　　　　　e. nose bridge, nose tip surgery

2. 阅读课文,完成翻译

(1) 我想咨询关于双眼皮手术的事项。

(2) 双眼皮全切手术可以打造自然的双眼皮,且效果持久。

(3) 双眼皮埋线手术是非侵入性的,且没有切口。

(4) 术后的两到四周内,肿胀和瘀青会消失。

(5) 我怎么样进行行术后护理?

(6) 术后48小时内用冰纱布垫敷眼镜和双颊。

(7) 你可以在小册子上找到所有关于术前和术后的注意事项。

Key 3-3

3. 阅读报告 掌握动态

Chinese Plastic Surgery Trends You Need To Know About

Recent studies by HSBC have predicted that Chinese plastic surgery markets will double in size by 2019. This would make it the third-largest in the world, after the United States and Brazil. By the end of 2019, it is expected to reach the size of 800 million yuan, which is around US $122 billion.

There are many popular surgeries in China, with things like double eyelid surgery, face slimming and calf slimming surgeries being some of the most popular. Lack of trust in Chinese hospitals and even private hospitals means that many Chinese consumers travel out of the country to undergo procedures, however the domestic market has seen tremendous growth in recent years.

In the next few years, the Chinese plastic surgery market is expected to boom even more than it already is. This is going to increase the intense competition between both international and domestic hospitals and surgeries, who are courting the increasing amount of mainlanders who wish to change their looks.

The Most Popular Types of Cosmetic Surgeries in China

Social media has increased the presence of different types of beauty to Chinese consumers. The specific types of surgeries that are becoming popular are suggesting what Chinese consumers value and what they consider to be beautiful.

The double eyelid surgeries are probably the most popular and the most widely known surgery for China. This procedure involves lifting up the eyelid in order to create the appearance of western eyelids. However, it's not just double eyelid surgeries, over 50% of cosmetic surgeries in China are focused on the eyes according to Mylike.

Another trend that is popular, especially amongst young men is calf slimming surgeries. In Asia, the long leg look is incredibly popular and this is why it is a popular surgery.

One Chinese plastic surgery trend is "lunch-break cosmetics". These are non-invasive surgeries such as Botox which can be done very quickly and the results are instant.

Aesthetic medicine is increasingly becoming the most popular form of Chinese plastic surgery. This category includes a variety of different treatments with the most popular being Botox. However, Allergan is the only company that has the exclusive right to distribute & market the product known as Botox, so be careful when marketing non-invasive procedures under the name botox!

A final type of popular surgery is the face slimming surgery. Many women want to emulate western features by slimming the face and creating a sharper chin. This has been popular for years in Asian countries and has finally caught on quite heavily in China as well.

China Plastic Surgery Trends: Age & Demographics

Those who undergo Chinese plastic surgery tend to be on the younger side compared to other countries. HSBC noted in its above-mentioned report that 80% of non-surgical procedures in the United States are done by those over the age of 35, but those younger than 35 make up the biggest portion in China.

As stated in the *China Daily,* "The younger generation (aged 20—35) are key to the market. Those aged under 28 were reportedly more than half of the 22 million consumers who went in for cosmetic procedures this year."

Similar to the people of ROK, many Chinese consumers who can afford it, give cosmetic surgery to friends and family as presents in their younger years. Even graduation presents can sometimes be cosmetic surgery, although they tend to fall into the non-permanent category.

While this may seem extreme in other countries, this is a commonplace occurrence in China. Often members of the older generation frown upon plastic surgery, so it makes sense that it is the younger generation is undergoing surgery.

Social media and increased information about surgical processes are considered to be the primary drivers of this trend. With many younger Chinese feeling that their looks are inadequate compared to the people, they see online it's no surprise plastic surgery is more popular among these younger generations. The launch of plastic surgery focused apps that we will discuss below have also helped educate users about how plastic surgery is done and the risks associated with it.

(*Source:* Tony DeGennaro, Dragon Social, 23 August 2019)

Video 3-9

II Extensive Learning【拓展学习　媒体动态】

The Chinese cosmetic surgery industry was valued at 495.3 billion yuan ($71.8 billion) in 2018, according to a report released on Thursday by cosmetic procedure platform GengMei (more beautiful in Chinese).

The report further found that the establishment of cosmetic procedure facilities increased by more than 10 percent in comparison with 2017 in most provinces.

About 22 million Chinese people underwent cosmetic procedures in 2018, and consumers under the age of 28 accounted for 54 percent of the total, the report said.

Those born after 2000 took an 8 percent share among consumers in 2018, and over-95s took 15 percent. Hyaluronic acid injection and double-eyelid surgeries were among the most popular procedures with young people, according to the report.

Read more from
China Daily, 2018

Read more 3-5

Ireland-based pharmaceutical giant Allergan is planning to increase investment in China and train more local medical cosmetic professionals, as the country's medical aesthetic industry booms and the sector is in urgent need of talents, said a senior executive.

"We are looking at training 5,800 medical cosmetic professionals, who have already got a medical license, in China this year," said Fan Jing, executive director of medical education at Allergan China.

Working with the Chinese Association of Plastics and Aesthetics, on June 13, Allergan China launched its first medical cosmetics course at its newly built innovation center in Chengdu, Southwest China's Sichuan province, to give medical professionals systematic training in areas such as anatomical basis, aesthetic evaluation, consumer communication and photography.

Read more from
China Daily, 2019

Read more 3-6

Section D

Projects in Practice【实践探索　行动项目】

1. Project 1

Psychological Evaluation：心理评估

Read the information about psychological evaluation below. Work with a partner and ask and answer the following questions.

Psychological Evaluation of Cosmetic Surgery Patients

With this growing interest and number of people seeking cosmetic procedures, it has also become important to evaluate the patient's motives and understand what they think plastic surgery can do for them. Unrealistic expectations or impure motives can lead to problems for both the individual undergoing the procedure, as well as the doctors involved in performing the surgery.

Here are some of the questions consultants can ask in order to be more aware of what to look for in patients for cosmetic surgery.

- What types of surgery are you considering?
- What specific features do you dislike?
- How long have you been thinking about having surgery?
- What caused you to begin thinking about it?
- Have you read articles about cosmetic surgery?
- Do you understand that the object of any cosmetic operation is improvement in appearance, not perfection?
- Is having surgery your idea or is someone else urging you to have it?
- Do you feel guilty or embarrassed about wanting the surgery?
- If you have the surgery, who do you think will be the happiest with the results?
- Do you have any preconceived idea of how you would like your nose, face, etc., to look? If yes, how?
- Have you spoken to your family of your desire for surgery? If no, do you mind if they know? If yes, what was their attitude?
- Have you spoken to your friends of your desire for surgery? If no, do you mind if they know? If yes, what was their attitude?
- Have you recently experienced any significant disappointment, sorrow, of loss of self-esteem?
- Any emotional crisis at home, work or in any relationship?
- Why did you wait until now to come in for surgery?

2. Project 2

Role Play:角色扮演

Work with a partner. Based on the text, adjust the dialogue by changing the customer demand and surgery. Act out the consultation.

Video 3-10

Section E

Self-assessment【进阶评估　自我超越】

1. Cooperative Learning Assessment

Please check your contribution to the group after the project is done.

	Superior (5)	Above Average (4)	Average (3)	Below Average (2)	Weak (1)
Understood what was required for the project					
Participated in the group discussion					
Helped the group to function well as a team					
Contributed useful ideas					
How much work was done					
Quality of completed work					
What could you improve upon next time?					
Your group members' comments					
Your group leader's comments					

2. Assessment of Your Study

Instructions:

(1) Read each statement in the table below and place a check mark in the column that best describes how well you can complete that task.

(2) Review your responses for each task. If you have checked five or more in the "Somewhat" and / or "No" columns, you may need to consider making greater efforts after class.

I can	Yes	Somewhat	No
Understand the main idea of the text			
Identify the major points, important facts and details, and vocabulary in the text			
Make inferences about what is implied in the text			
Recognize the organization and purpose of the text			
Remember the new words and expressions			
Speak on the topic effectively			
Employ search strategy to gain information to address the project			
Refer to appropriate resources to deal with the project			

3. Personal Development

Instruction:

Completing this section will help you make informed practicing decisions. Please identify your strengths and the areas that you need to develop or strengthen and record them below.

STRENGTHS:
I am confident that I can...
(1)
(2)
(3)
AREAS FOR IMPROVEMENT:
I would like to improve my ability to...
(1)
(2)
(3)

4. Say What You Want to Say

(1) What are the possible risks and side effects of rhinoplasty surgery?

(2) If customer has unrealistic expectations of cosmetic surgery, what would you do as cosmetic staff?

Unit 4   Cosmetics Products

美妆产品

🩺 Section A

Warm-up Activity【精致生活　匠心呵护】

1. Write Down the Top 10 Cosmetic Brand and Try to Properly Pronounce Them

1 LANCÔME ✿ PARIS	2 L'ORÉAL PARIS	3 ESTĒE LAUDER	4 OLAY	5 MAYBELLINE NEW YORK
6 SK-II	7 innisfree	8 佰草集 INOHERO	9 LANEIGE	10 CLINIQUE

2. Match the Chinese Phrases with Right English Expressions

(1) 面霜   a. essence

(2) 洗面奶   b. cream

(3) 精华   c. toner

(4) 爽肤水   d. cleanser

(5) 眼霜   e. lotion

(6) 乳液   f. fragrance free

(7) 面膜   g. allergy

(8) 防晒霜   h. eye cream

(9) 不含香精   i. facial mask

(10) 过敏   j. sunscreen

🩺 Section B

Ⅰ Dialogue: Understand Products【有依有据　读出真谛】

1. Cosmetic Labeling Reading

Cosmetic (美容的) products are applied to the human body for the purposes of cleaning, beautifying, promoting attractiveness or changing its appearance. They play an essential role in all stages of our life.

For customers' safety and confidence, cosmetic industry is required to provide important information about cosmetic products through labeling (用标签标明).

Label is a written, printed or graphic (图像的) display of information on the package (包裹) of a cosmetic product. Label should convey (传达) its information in a manner that is easily read and understandable because the information needs to be communicated to a customer.

Required Information That Must Appear on A Label

Despite different cosmetic labeling regulations (规定) across the world, there's certain information that is so essential that it's required to appear on a label by most countries and regions (地区). These include:

(1) product identity (本体)；

(2) name and address of business；

(3) net quantity；

(4) warning statements；

(5) ingredients (成分).

Labels	标签	Significance
identity	真实属性	indicate the nature and use of the product
name and address of business	生产者的名称和地址	tell who is responsible for the product
net quantity	净含量	declare the actual quantity
warning statements	安全警告用语	help customers use the product safely
ingredients	成分表(成分按加入量的降序列出)	for people who have allergies (过敏反应) so that they may avoid ingredients to which they are allergic (过敏的).

2. Other Labeling Information

Although some countries, such as U.S. and Canada, do not require cosmetic manufacturers (制造商) to print shelf life or expiration (截止) dates on the labels, E.U. and China require manufactures to print either shelf life or expiration dates on the labels. A "best used before the end of" or a "period after opening" shows for how long the product may be kept or used.

Information on cosmetic labeling, including claims (声称), must be truthful and not false or misleading (误导的). Here are some claims that are common on the packages of cosmetic products and customers need to be cautious about:

(1) alcohol free；

(2) cruelty (残忍) free / not tested on animals；

(3) hypoallergenic (不会导致过敏反应的)；

(4) organic (有机的).

3. Cosmetic Product Consultation

Proper labeling helps customers make informed choices (在信息充足的情况下做出选择) about cosmetic products. Sometimes customers may have difficulties understanding all the labels. Therefore, it's cosmetic professionals' job to communicate all the important information on labels to customers. Here is an example.

Video 3-11

(Ms. Zhao is interested a cleanser displayed at the front desk at the beauty salon. She asks the beautician about the cleanser.)

A: Beauty Consultant   B: Ms. Zhao

A: Hi, Ms. Zhao. How are you feeling after the facial treatment?

B: I feel refreshed now, thank you.

A: Here is your bill.

B: OK. I'll use Alipay. Wait, what is it on display?

A: It's a cleanser. Our salon is teaming up this brand, Elta MD. It's a Swiss-American brand. It's famous for its cleanser.

B: I'm looking for a new cleanser right now. However, it's hard to find one suitable for my combination and sensitive skin.

A: Apparently this cleanser is a good fit for you. Look, it's sensitivity-free and oil-free. And it's pH-balanced. It thoroughly (彻底地) cleanses your face without irritating (刺激) your skin.

B: This is good news. Can you have a look at the ingredients? Does it contain any toxic (有毒的) ingredients?

A: From what I see, all these ingredients are gentle yet effective.

B: I'm relieved. Thank you for explaining. To be honest, it's so difficult to understand these ingredients.

A: I feel you. Actually these ingredients are listed by INCI names. You can look them up online.

B: Ok. Thanks for the advice. How much is it?

A: It's 168 yuan for 207 mL. It's a very affordable price.

B: I'll have one. Here is my QR code.

A: OK. Thank you.

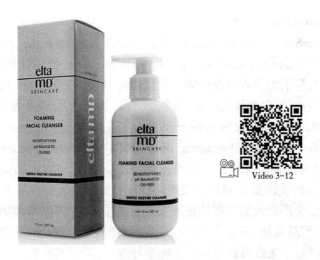

Video 3-12

Ⅱ Notes【说文解字　名词注释】

1. Vocabulary Table

Vocabulary 3-4

Words & Expressions	Part of Speech	Meaning in Text
cosmetic	*adj.*	美容的
label	*v.*	用标签标明
graphic	*adj.*	绘画的;绘图的;图像的
package	*n.*	包;包裹
convey	*v.*	传达;表达;传递
regulation	*n.*	规则;规章;规定;制度
region	*n.*	地区
identity	*n.*	本体
ingredient	*n.*	成分
allergy	*n.*	过敏反应
allergic	*adj.*	过敏的
manufacturer	*n.*	生产商;制造商
expiration	*n.*	告终;期满;截止
claim	*n.*	声称
misleading	*adj.*	误导性的;迷惑性的;欺骗性的
cruelty	*n.*	残暴;残忍;残酷
hypoallergenic	*adj.*	(化妆品、耳环等)不会导致过敏反应的
organic	*adj.*	有机的
make informed choices	*phr.*	在信息充足的情况下做出选择
thoroughly	*adv.*	彻底地
irritate	*v.*	刺激(身体部位);使发痒;使疼痛
toxic	*adj.*	有毒的

2. Useful Knowledge

(1) Cosmetic products are applied to the human body for the purposes of cleaning, beautifying, promoting attractiveness or changing its appearance. 使用化妆品的目的是为了清洁或美化身体,提升吸引力或者改变外表。化妆品是一个广义的概念,包含护肤品、彩妆品、洗护发品、头发定型产品、染发烫发产品、香氛类产品、沐浴产品、洗手液等。

(2) Despite different cosmetic labeling regulations across the world, there's certain information that is so essential that it's required to appear on a label by most countries and regions. 尽管各国的美容护肤化妆品对标签的管理各不相同,但绝大部分国家和地区都要求标签上必须标注特定的重要信息。如:美国食品和药物管理局(FDA)要求必须在标签上标注出产品真实属性、净含量、成分表、生产者的名称和地址和安全警告用语;中国国家市场监督管理总局则要求在标签上标注出产品名称、净含量、成分表、生产者的名称和地址、安全警告用语、保质期、企业的生产许可证号、卫生许可证号和产品标准好等。

(3) shelf life or expiration dates:限期使用日期或有效期。

(4) best used before the end of:请在标注日期前使用。属于限期使用日期的表达方式一种。

(5) period after opening(PAO)：开瓶后的使用日期，属于限期使用日期的表达方式一种。

(6) claim：化妆品标签上的宣传词。宣传词不受监管，也无须化妆品企业提供证据证明真实性，所以顾客需要警惕。

(7) cruelty free / not tested on animals：零残忍，即不在动物身上测试化妆品。鉴于动物伦理的原因，目前，国外许多国家和地区都已相继颁布了禁止在动物身上测试化妆品的条例。欧盟禁止销售采用动物做实验品的美容产品。但我国目前仍然进行动物试验。这导致了许多欧美化妆品企业直接放弃中国市场。同样，中国化妆品企业产品也无法进入欧美市场。目前，中国正在探索用其他技术手段替代动物实验。

(8) hypoallergenic：低过敏性的。这是常见的化妆品企业印在产品标签上的宣传词。宣传词不受监管，也无须化妆品企业提供证据证明真实性，所以顾客需要警惕。

(9) organic：有机的。这是常见的化妆品企业印在产品标签上的宣传词。宣传词不受监管，也无须化妆品企业提供证据证明真实性，所以顾客需要警惕。

(10) International Nomenclature Cosmetic Ingredient(INCI)：国际化妆品原料命名。在中国大陆境内销售的化妆品，都需要在产品包装上明确标示产品中添加的所有成分的中文标准名称。

Section C

Ⅰ Enhanced Learning【深度学习　品质保障】

1. 护肤产品，选词填空

| hydration SPF PA concentrated toners |
| nourish balance sunburn balance exfoliate |

(1) There're two types of _____ available in the market: natural and alcohol-based.

(2) Moisturizing is important in skin care routine because it ensures _____.

(3) Serum is highly _____. You only need to use a few drops to cover your face. Remember, less is more.

(4) Applying sheet mask is an effective and convenient way to _____ skin.

(5) When choosing a sunscreen, consider _____. The higher the number, the longer the protection.

2. 阅读课文，翻译填空
(1) 这是您的账单。
(2) 这款爽肤水适合混合型皮肤。
(3) 这款洗面奶能彻底清洗面部，但不刺激皮肤。
(4) 成分温和且有效。
(5) 这款产品价格合理。

Key 3-4

3. 阅读博文,掌握动态

Six Ingredients to Look for in Your Skincare

With the recent rise in attention to skincare, nowadays it seems like everyone has some unique solution when it comes to skin problems. With all the different ingredients out there in skin products, I wanted to investigate what we really should and shouldn't be putting on our faces. Here is a list of the top six ingredients you should look for in your skincare!

Salicylic Acid

This is probably an ingredient you've heard of before. Salicylic acid is known for its exfoliant properties. It is great for the gentle removal of dead skin to leave you glowing like a goddess. Salicylic acid is also good for acne treatment.

Caffeine

Just as a cup of coffee wakes you up in the morning, caffeine in your skincare does the same thing. It works to stimulate your skin and make you appear less tired. Look for caffeine as an ingredient in your eye creams in particular. Caffeine also works to calm inflammation and irritation.

Coconut Oil

As an ingredient, coconut oil is great for helping your skin create a moisture barrier, meaning it helps to lock moisturizing products in. Look for coconut oil in your moisturizers and face washes.

Cucumber

Cucumber is high in vitamin C, an ingredient known to help rejuvenate tired skin and while also hydrating.

Rose

Not only does this ingredient make your skin products smell amazing, it also is amazing for your skin! Rose not only works as an anti-redness agent, it also calms the skin. Rose is especially good for acne-prone skin, as it carries antibacterial properties that work to reduce acne and prevent scarring.

Green Tea

Green tea actually can work as a cancer-fighting ingredient for your skin. It helps promote the renewal of DNA and works to protect you against UV rays. Because of this it also is great at slowing the signs of aging! Look for this ingredient in your night creams, or serums.

II Extensive Learning【拓展学习 媒体动态】

We are all familiar with Western and Korean cosmetics brands such as Lancôme, Maybelline, Innisfree, Etude House and so on. But China also has their own domestic cosmetics brands that are worth checking out! The Chinese cosmetics industry is currently on the rise as the Chinese government continues to offer their support to domestic brands and work to dispel the notion that all foreign brands are superior. Here are some of the most well known cosmetics brands from China, and their best selling products. Let's take a look!

Chando

Chando was established in Shanghai in 2009 and is one of the most successful domestic cosmetics brands in China, with endorsements from the likes of Fan Bingbing and other Chinese celebrities. They operate throughout mainland China and also have retail locations in the USA, Russia and Britain.

Read more from
Baopals, 2018

Read more 3-7

Brands are teaming up with internet celebrities, fashionistas and beauty experts to engage with potential clients, drive sales

Despite being the founder of Alibaba Group, the world's largest e-commerce company by transaction volume, Jack Ma doesn't seem to know much about selling lipstick.

In a video that went viral ahead of last year's Nov. 11 promotion—a global shopping festival established by the online retailer—Ma pitted himself against Li Jiaqi, a broadcaster known for endorsing and selling lipsticks through live broadcasts and short-form videos. In the allotted time, Li sold 100 times as many lipsticks as the business guru.

Read more from
China Daily, 2019

Read more 3-8

🩺 **Section D**

Projects in Practice【实践探索　行动项目】

1. Project 1

Cosmetic Label Reading:化妆品标签阅读

Read the back label of a Burt's Bees product and answer the following questions.

(1) What is this product?

(2) What can the product do to skin?

(3) How can the product be applied?

(4) Can the product be put near fire?

(5) Does the product contain glycerin?

(6) Which ingredient is the second largest amount?

(7) Has the product be tested on animals?

(8) How long can the product be used once it's open?

(9) Where is the product made?

(10) What's the name and address of the manufacture?

rosewater toner

This natural toner is developed with a botanical blend of cleansing and softening ingredients to gently remove lingering traces of cleanser and any trapped dirt, oil and make-up. Formulated with Rosewater Extract, Glycerin and Aloe, your skin is left feeling naturally clean and refreshed.

Directions: After cleansing and/or exfoliating, moisten a cotton pad with toner and apply to face and neck using upward movements, avoiding the eye area.

CAUTION: FLAMMABLE. Keep away from flame and high heat.

lotion tonifiante à l'eau de rose

Faite d'un mélange d'ingrédients nettoyants et adoucissants de sources végétales, cette lotion tonifiante naturelle déloge délicatement les résidus de produit nettoyant, de maquillage, de saleté et de sébum. À base d'extrait d'eau de rose, de glycérine et d'aloès, ce produit procurera à votre peau une sensation de propreté et de fraicheur naturelles.

Mode d'emploi : Après le nettoyage et/ou le gommage de la peau, imbiber un coton à démaquiller de lotion et appliquer sur le visage et le cou en effectuant des mouvements vers le haut. Éviter le contour des yeux.

ATTENTION : INFLAMMABLE. Tenir à l'écart des flammes et des sources de chaleur élevée.

Ingredients / Ingrédients : aqua (water, eau), alcohol denat., glycerin, rosa damascena flower extract, aloe barbadensis leaf juice, hamamelis virginiana water, maltodextrin, yucca schidigera leaf/root/stem extract, centaurea cyanus flower extract, alcohol, sodium citrate, citric acid, potassium sorbate, sodium benzoate, phenoxyethanol, linalool, geraniol, citronellol

Made in USA • Fabriqué aux États-Unis • Dist. for/pour : BURT'S BEES, Inc. Durham, NC 27701, US • BURT'S BEES Canada, Brampton, ON L6W 4V3, CA CBEE (Europe) Ltd. Richmond, TW9 1SE, UK

2. Project 2

Role Play:角色扮演

(Mrs. Richards is at a cosmetics counter in a department store. She asks a beauty assistant for a recommendation about sunscreen.)

A: Beauty Assistant   B: Mrs. Richards

A: Hello, madam. How can I help you today?

B: I'm looking for a sunscreen for my little kids. I'm on the summer break. We're going to Bali soon.

A: OK. It's important to keep children's skin protected from an early age.

B: I need the best and safest sunscreens.

A: Sure. How about this baby sunscreen?

B: Does it provide protection against UVA and UVB?

A: Yes. Actually it goes the extra mile with this UVA & UVB protecting sunscreen for your baby.

B: Really?

A: Yes. See the SPF number? It's 50.

B: What does this mean?

A: SPF stands for sun protection factor. The higher the SPF number, the longer the protection against UVB rays.

B: Oh, I see. UVB causes sunburn, right?

A: Correct.

B: What's this? PA＋＋＋?

A: PA stands for the Protection Grade of UVA. The more "＋", the higher level of protection against UVA rays. PA＋＋＋ means great protection against UVA.

B: I've never seen this on American sunscreen.

A: It's because PA is established by the Japanese. Therefore, it's often seen on Asian sunscreens.

B: What damage do UVA rays cause?

A: UVA rays penetrate deeper into skin. Therefore, they're the main cause for skin cancer.

B: Oh my God. It's terrible.

A: This sunscreen is fragrance free and chemical free. It's suitable for sensitive skin. Moreover, it's water and sweat resistant, which is perfect for the beach trip.

B: Great! My kids can use it.

A: Yes.

Video 3-13

🩺 Section E

Self-assessment【进阶评估 自我超越】

1. Cooperative Learning Assessment

Please check your contribution to the group after the project is done.

	Superior (5)	Above Average (4)	Average (3)	Below Average (2)	Weak (1)
Understood what was required for the project					
Participated in the group discussion					
Helped the group to function well as a team					
Contributed useful ideas					
How much work was done					
Quality of completed work					
What could you improve upon next time?					
Your group members' comments					
Your group leader's comments					

2. Assessment of Your Study

Instructions:

(1) Read each statement in the table below and place a check mark in the column that best describes how well you can complete that task.

(2) Review your responses for each task. If you have checked five or more in the "Somewhat" and / or "No" columns, you may need to consider making greater efforts after class.

I can	Yes	Somewhat	No
Understand the main idea of the text			
Identify the major points, important facts and details, and vocabulary in the text			
Make inferences about what is implied in the text			
Recognize the organization and purpose of the text			
Remember the new words and expressions			
Speak on the topic effectively			
Employ search strategy to gain information to address the project			
Refer to appropriate resources to deal with the project			

3. Personal Development

Instruction:

Completing this section will help you make informed practicing decisions. Please identify your strengths and the areas that you need to develop or strengthen and record them below.

STRENGTHS: I am confident that I can...
(1)
(2)
(3)
AREAS FOR IMPROVEMENT: I would like to improve my ability to...
(1)
(2)
(3)

4. Say What You Want to Say

(1) What should customers look for when they're buying sunscreen?

(2) What's your "holy grail" cosmetic product?

Unit 5　Nail Care
美甲护理

Video 3–14

Section A

Warm-up Activity【启动大脑　得心应手】

1. Combine the Words from the Box to Create Some Correct Expressions About Nail Care

> nail clear cuticle clippers gel artificial polish clippers buffer pusher
> trimmer whitener pencil coat varnish remover tips file acrylic dryer

2. Work with a Partner and Take It in Turns to Be the Consultant and the Customer and Fill in the Customer Card

Good communication with customers is essential. You need to understand why the customer came to your salon and why she / he is paying you to do her / his nails.

Your job is to identify the customer's needs and fulfill them. The consultation is your first opportunity to educate and impress the customer. The "Customer Card" is an ideal method for guiding this conversation and gathering essential information.

Customer Card / Consultation Form

Name:＿＿＿＿＿＿＿＿＿＿＿＿＿　Birthday:＿＿＿＿＿＿＿＿＿＿＿＿＿＿

Address:

Mobile phone:＿＿＿＿＿＿＿＿＿　Email:＿＿＿＿＿＿＿＿＿＿＿＿＿＿＿

What services brought you into the salon?

＿＿＿＿＿＿＿＿＿＿＿＿＿＿＿＿＿＿＿＿＿＿＿＿＿＿＿＿＿＿＿＿＿＿＿＿＿

Do you have any condition that could affect service choices, such as allergies, diabetes or other circulation disorders, slow healing, sensitivity to any cosmetic ingredients? Please explain.

＿＿＿＿＿＿＿＿＿＿＿＿＿＿＿＿＿＿＿＿＿＿＿＿＿＿＿＿＿＿＿＿＿＿＿＿＿

What services have you enjoyed in the past?

＿＿＿＿＿＿＿＿＿＿＿＿＿＿＿＿＿＿＿＿＿＿＿＿＿＿＿＿＿＿＿＿＿＿＿＿＿

How did you find out about us?

＿＿＿＿＿＿＿＿＿＿＿＿＿＿＿＿＿＿＿＿＿＿＿＿＿＿＿＿＿＿＿＿＿＿＿＿＿

Are you preparing for a special occasion?

_____

What is your activity level/occupation?

_____

Do you play any sports that take a toll on hands or feet?

_____

What products do you use on your hands, nails, and feet?

_____

Do you have any special concerns you would like to discuss?

_____

Additional information:

_____

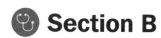 Section B

I Dialogue: Nail Services【玉指纤纤　美丽无限】

(Ms. Fang is a regular guest of the nail salon. The beautician is giving her a manicure.)

A: Beautician　　B: Ms. Fang

A: Hello, Ms. Fang. What would you like to have today?

B: Hello. I'd like to have my regular (固定的) treatment, the basic manicure.

A: OK. Sit down please. Let me first remove (去除) the old nail polish (指甲油).

B: Sure.

A: What shape would you like? Round, square, squared oval (方圆形), oval (椭圆形), or stiletto (尖形)?

B: Squared oval, please.

A: OK. Now soak your hands in the warm water. After that, I'll treat your cuticles (表皮).

B: Alright. Please push them back gently.

A: Of course. Trust me. While I'm massaging your hands, you can think about what nail polish color you'd like. Here's the color card.

B: I'd like to try new color this time.

A: How about this neon (霓虹的) purple? It's bright and loud.

B: Yes, it's such a unique color. I'll try this color.

A: OK. I'll paint two coats of this nail polish when the base coat dries. After that, I'll finish your manicure (美甲) with the top coat and let it dry for 15 minutes.

B: It sounds great. Thank you.

A: You're welcome.

Video 3-15

(Ms. Lin's wedding is round the corner. She comes to the nail salon to do a wedding manicure.)

A: Beautician   B: Ms. Lin

A: Good afternoon, Ms. Lin. How are you doing today?

B: Good afternoon. I'd like to do a wedding manicure today. I'm going to marry this Saturday.

A: Congratulations!

B: Thank you.

A: What type of manicure would you like for your wedding? The classic French manicure or dramatic acrylic nail (水晶指甲)?

B: I prefer French manicure. I want my manicure simple and clean.

A: OK. What nail polish color would you like?

B: What's your recommendation?

A: The color you choose should complement (衬托出) your overall look. Neutral (无色的) or nude (裸色的) always look clean and elegant (典雅的).

B: I'll choose nude. It goes with (伴随) everything.

A: OK.

(After an hour)

A: All right, it's done.

B: How much is it?

A: It's 188 yuan. We offer you, the bride-to-be (准新娘) a 20% discount (折扣). We wish you a wonderful wedding ceremony this Saturday.

B: Thank you very much.

Ⅱ Notes【说文解字　名词注释】

1. Vocabulary Table

Vocabulary 3-5

Words & Expressions	Part of Speech	Meaning in Text
regular	*adj.*	经常使用的;固定的
remove	*v.*	(用化学品)去除;洗掉(污渍)
polish	*n.*	指甲油
oval	*n.*	椭圆形
cuticle	*n.*	(手指甲根部的)表皮;护膜
neon	*adj.*	霓虹的
manicure	*n.*	修指甲;美甲;手部护理
complement	*v.*	使(优点)突出;衬托出
neutral	*adj.*	灰暗的;素净的;无色的
nude	*adj.*	裸色的
elegant	*adj.*	典雅的;雅致的;优美的
go with	*phr.*	伴随
discount	*n.*	折扣

2. Useful Knowledge

(1) manicure：手指甲护理。和它相对的是Pedicure，脚指甲护理。

(2) Round, square, squared oval, oval, or stiletto? 指甲形状要圆形，方形，方圆形，椭圆形，还是尖形？圆形适合短指甲的人或指甲长得矮矮胖胖的类型；方形指甲适合指甲较长、面积较大的指甲，可以从视觉上收窄指甲，让指甲显得比实际上小；方圆形美甲形状优雅大方，适合大多数人；椭圆形指甲外形最为优雅，能掩饰纤细或宽大甲面的缺点，椭圆形指尖能让指甲显得纤细修长；尖形美甲形状最适合搭配水晶甲或艺术美甲，适合有长指甲的人。

(3) It's bright and loud. 这个颜色明亮、显眼。loud表示颜色大胆、明艳。

(4) French manicure：法式甲。传统的法式指甲，是利用白色指甲油，在指甲前端画出有如微笑般的圆弧形。

(5) acrylic nails：水晶甲。水晶甲是一种美甲，是目前多种美甲工艺中最受欢迎的一种，其特点是能从视觉上改变手指形状，给人以修长感，从而弥补手形不美的遗憾。

Section C

I Enhanced Learning【深度学习　指尖艺术】

1. 阅读课文 完成填空

(1) I'll _____ two coats of this _____ when the _____ dries.
当底油干了以后我会涂两层指甲油。

(2) I'll finish your _____ with the _____.
亮油是你美甲的最后一步。

(3) I'd like to do a _____.
我想做一个新娘美甲。

(4) The classic _____ or dramatic _____?
经典的法式甲还是引人注目的水晶甲？

(5) We _____ you a _____.
我们给你打八折。

2. 阅读课文，翻译填空

(1) 我想做我的常规项目，基础美甲。

(2) 我先卸掉旧指甲油。

(3) 把手浸在温水中。

(4) 你想涂什么颜色的指甲油？

(5) 中性色或裸色看上去干净、优雅。

Key 3–5

3. 阅读博文,掌握动态

The 8 Major Dos and Don'ts of Bridal Nails

Picking your wedding day shade and type of manicure is only half the battle when it comes to getting your bridal nails perfectly polished before your wedding. There are going to be a lot of people looking at your hands to catch a glimpse of that pretty new ring (and a lot of high-definition close-up shots taken by your photographer), so read the below to prevent any major bridal-nail blunders.

(1) Don't get a gel or dip manicure more than a few days in advance.

Gel and dip manicures were one of the best things to happen to bridal nails. Instant dry time and chip-free for weeks? Yep—it's literally a dream come true. But after a few days, both types start to lose their luster. Get them done only one or two days before your wedding to avoid any wear and tear by the time your actual wedding day rolls around.

(2) Do test multiple shades.

You try on more than one dress (most of the time), so why shouldn't you try on more than one polish for your wedding day nails? Keep in mind that certain shades look better on different skin tones.

(3) Don't buy only one bottle of polish.

If you always prefer polish, once you've found your perfect shade, stock up: one for the salon, one for your wedding day emergency kit and one to pack in your honeymoon bag. When you need to fix a chipped nail fast, you'll be happy you spent the extra cash.

(4) Do remember to maintain your nails at home.

If you know you're an avid nail biter, make a conscious effort to kick the habit in the months leading up to your wedding. Also, avoid peeling broken nails and picking at hangnail—that's how infections start.

(5) Don't get too adventurous with nail art for the first time.

We're all for a fun nail design, but if you're not usually a "glitter and appliqué" kind of girl, your wedding day isn't the time to experiment with nail art. Go for a tried-and-true shade or a timeless look (like French tips, for instance) for your bridal nails instead.

(6) Do remember to bring your own bottle to the salon.

Even if the dreamy color you picked is a salon staple, it's always a good idea to come prepared with your own bottle of polish just in case your color isn't there or the bottle they have is old. It's better to be safe than sorry.

(7) Don't freak out over a chipped nail.

Speaking of chipping, it's bound to happen with a polish manicure, but we promise it isn't the end of the world. Use the tip of the brush to fill in the hole, then let the polish dry for 30 seconds. Next, brush on a second coat of polish and finish with a thin clear top coat.

(8) Do moisturize your hands (always).

It's amazing what a little hand cream can do for your pictures—seriously. For instantly younger looking hands, massage cream into your cuticles and knuckles before your photographer takes close-ups of your bouquet or ring.

Ⅱ Extensive Learning【拓展学习　媒体动态】

A woman has been forced to have surgery after getting her nails done at a salon.

The woman shared her story on Facebook about the experience she had at a nail salon on the NSW Central Coast where she was a regular.

"I've been happy with my nails for years and never had any problems, however after my last infill a couple of weeks ago my finger tip started swelling up and was quite painful about a week after my infill," she said.

She said the pain got so bad she ended up taking herself to hospital in Wyong on July 28, and ended up staying there the whole day until she was sent home in the afternoon with antibiotics, and a referral to see a specialist doctor.

Read more from
Yahoo News Australia, 2019

Read more 3-9

Every girl likes a little nail polish. In fact, a manicure can be an easy way to give yourself a boost.

But if you're going to a salon to have it done, you need to be sure you won't walk out with more than you bargained for, like an infection.

"American Idol"'s Paula Abdul made headlines earlier this year when an infection from a bad manicure caused her to lose her thumbnail.

Allure magazine's editor-in-chief, Linda Wells, visits The Early Show on Tuesday to offer some tips on how you can prevent that from happening to you. Also, she will talk about the latest trends in length, shapes and colors for fall.

Read more from
CBS News, 2004

Read more 3-10

Section D

Projects in Practice 【实践探索　行动项目】

1. Project 1

Conversation: 沟通交流

Give some professional advice to your customers. What to do if:

(1) the customer would like to have beautiful nails；

(2) the nails need to strengthen；

(3) the varnish doesn't last long enough；

(4) the customer bites her nails；

(5) the customer is getting married in two days.

Video 3-16

2. Project 2

Role Play: 角色扮演

The beautician is explaining pedicure to Miss Liu.

A: Beautician　　B: Miss Liu

A: Hello, madam. How are you doing?

B: Hello. I heard you offer pedicure in here as well.

A: Yes, we do cosmetic treatments for feet.

B: What is included in the treatment?

A: Our basic pedicure begins with soaking your feet in hot water. After cleansing and scrubbing the feet, we will trim and file the nails and remove the cuticles. Then we will massage your feet. Finally, nail polished will be applied if you'd like.

B: Oh, I see. Will the pedicure help me get glowing smooth feet?

A: Absolutely! Your feet will look flawless.

B: How much would it cost?

A: Our basic pedicure costs 100 yuan.

B: Alright. Can I have one now?

A: Sure.

B: Perfect. Thank you.

Section E

Self-assessment【进阶评估　自我超越】

1. Cooperative Learning Assessment

Please check your contribution to the group after the project is done.

	Superior (5)	Above Average (4)	Average (3)	Below Average (2)	Weak (1)
Understood what was required for the project					
Participated in the group discussion					
Helped the group to function well as a team					
Contributed useful ideas					
How much work was done					
Quality of completed work					
What could you improve upon next time?					
Your group members' comments					
Your group leader's comments					

2. Assessment of Your Study

Instructions:

(1) Read each statement in the table below and place a check mark in the column that best describes how well you can complete that task.

(2) Review your responses for each task. If you have checked five or more in the "Somewhat" and / or "No" columns, you may need to consider making greater efforts after class.

I can	Yes	Somewhat	No
Understand the main idea of the text			
Identify the major points, important facts and details, and vocabulary in the text			
Make inferences about what is implied in the text			
Recognize the organization and purpose of the text			
Remember the new words and expressions			
Speak on the topic effectively			
Employ search strategy to gain information to address the project			
Refer to appropriate resources to deal with the project			

3. Personal Development

Instruction:

Completing this section will help you make informed practicing decisions. Please identify your strengths and the areas that you need to develop or strengthen and record them below.

STRENGTHS:		
I am confident that I can...		
(1)		
(2)		
(3)		
AREAS FOR IMPROVEMENT:		
I would like to improve my ability to...		
(1)		
(2)		
(3)		

4. Say What You Want to Say

(1) If a kid would like to have a gel manicure, what would you do as a beautician?

(2) If a kid would like to have a gel manicure, what would you do as a parent?

Chapter 4

Child Care

幼儿照护

Unit 1　Teaching Kids About the Flu
流感预防

Section A

Video 4-1

Warm-up Activity【听歌记词　规范洗手】

1. Listen to the *Happy Handwashing Song* and Try to Get the Lyrics（Video 4-1）

_____

_____

_____

_____

_____

2. **Find and Circle the Eight Words in the Puzzle Below**

hygiene	soap
warm water	germs
wash hands	health
disease	scrub

Hand Washing Word Search

Find and circle the eight words in the puzzle below.

hygiene	soap
warm water	germs
wash hands	health
disease	scrub

```
w  o  g  q  s  w  w  n  d  l  e  b
a  s  d  l  a  l  a  m  w  t  n  m
s  g  o  y  g  e  r  m  s  h  e  n
h  r  m  a  h  w  m  j  t  e  i  h
h  u  x  k  b  s  w  d  o  a  g  e
a  y  d  i  s  e  a  s  e  g  y  a
n  a  t  e  c  e  t  y  d  s  h  l
d  m  s  h  r  a  e  b  o  h  q  t
s  l  i  q  u  i  r  o  d  m  g  h
d  i  g  b  b  a  l  p  a  o  s  w
```

Key 4-1

ESP Course for Students of
Health Science

医疗通识英语

Section B

Ⅰ Know About the Flu【知己知彼　远离流感】

Influenza (flu, 流感) is a contagious (传染性的) respiratory (呼吸的) illness caused by influenza viruses (病毒). It can cause mild to severe illness. Serious outcomes of flu infection (感染) can result in hospitalization or death. Some people, such as older people, young children, and people with certain health conditions, are at high risk of serious flu complications (并发症).

Flu seasons are unpredictable (不可预知的) in a number of ways. Although widespread flu activity occurs every year, the timing, severity, and duration of it depend on many factors, including which flu viruses are spreading, the number of people who are susceptible (亦受影响的) to the circulating flu viruses, and how similar vaccine (疫苗) viruses are to the flu viruses that are causing illness. The timing of flu can vary (改变) from season to season. In the United States, seasonal flu activity most commonly peaks (达到最高值) between December and March, but flu viruses can cause illness from early October to late May. Flu viruses are thought to spread mainly from person to person through coughs and sneezes (打喷嚏) of infected (已感染的) people. Less often, a person also might get the flu by touching a surface or object (物体) that has flu virus on it and then touching their own mouth, eyes, or nose. Influenza causes more hospitalizations among young children than any other vaccine-preventable disease.

General Information to Share with Children

(1) Germs (细菌) can make you sick. People can pass colds and flu through germs.

(2) Germs are everywhere. They are so small that you cannot see them without a microscope (显微镜).

(3) Cover your mouth and nose with a tissue (纸巾) when you cough or sneeze so you don't pass germs on to others. Throw the tissue in the trash after you use it.

(4) Wash your hands the right way to get rid of germs and lower the chance of spreading germs. Wash your hands often with soap and water, especially after you cough or sneeze. Use alcohol-based hand rubs or wipes (湿巾纸) when soap and water are not available (可得到的).

(5) Don't touch your eyes, nose, or mouth until your hands are clean because germs spread that way. Keeping your hands clean is one of the best ways to keep from getting sick and spreading illness.

Wash hands:

① after you cough or sneeze；

② after using the toilet；

③ after you play outside；

④ after shaking hands with other people；

⑤ after you touch animals, including your pet；

⑥ before you eat or touch food.

General Information to Share with Children About How Flu Spreads

(1) The flu spreads mostly from person to person through the coughs and sneezes of people who are sick with the flu. You may also get sick by touching something with flu viruses on it and then touching your mouth or nose.

(2) Tell children to let an adult know if they feel sick.

Ⅱ Notes【说文解字　名词注释】

1. Vocabulary Table

Vocabulary 4-1

Words & Expressions	Part of Speech	Meaning in Text
influenza（flu）	*n.*	流感
contagious	*adj.*	传染性的；会蔓延的
respiratory	*adj.*	呼吸的
virus	*n.*	病毒
infection	*n.*	感染；传染
complication	*n.*	并发症
unpredictable	*adj.*	不可预测的；无法预知的
susceptible	*adj.*	易受影响的
vaccine	*n.*	疫苗
vary	*v.*	变化；改变
peak	*v.*	达到高峰；达到最高值
sneeze	*v*	打喷嚏
infected	*adj.*	感染的
object	*n.*	事物；物体
germ	*n.*	细菌
microscope	*n.*	显微镜
tissue paper	*n.*	纸巾
wipe	*n.*	湿巾纸
available	*adj.*	可得到的；可利用的

2. Useful Knowledge

(1) influenza (flu), it is an illness which is similar to a bad cold but more serious. It often makes you feel very weak and make your muscles hurt.

常见跟 flu 相关的表达：bird flu 禽流感；flu virus 流感病毒；flu vaccine 流感疫苗；have the flu 得了流感，患流感。

(2) sneeze 表示"打喷嚏"的意思。感冒了老打喷嚏，我们就可以说：I caught a cold and sneezed a lot.

If someone sneeze, you may say "Bless you. (愿主保佑 你)" And if someone says "Bless you." when you sneeze, don't forget to respond "Thank you."

(3) cold symptoms：感冒症状。感冒常见的症状有

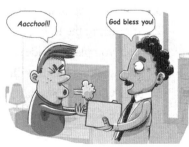

流鼻涕、打喷嚏、鼻塞、嗓子痛、头痛、咳嗽、发烧，这些症状的表达你都知道吗？

I've got a cold. / I've got a bad cold. 我感冒了 / 我重感冒。

I've got a runny nose. / My nose is running. 我流鼻涕。

I can't stop sneezing. 我不停滴打喷嚏。

I have a stuffy nose. 我鼻塞。

I've got a sore throat. 我嗓子疼。

I've got a very bad headache. / This headache is killing me. 我头痛死了。

I've been coughing day and night. 我咳嗽不停。

I've got a temperature. / I'm running a high fever. 我发烧了。

(4) germ (usually pl.): 细菌；病菌。

Dirty hands can be a breeding ground for germs. 脏手会滋生病菌。

(5) available：可获得的；可购得的；可找到的。

Resource 4-1

available resources / facilities 可利用的资源 / 设备。

readily / freely / publicly / generally available：容易 / 免费 / 让公众 / 普遍得到的。

This was the only room available. 这是唯一可用的房间。

We'll send you a copy as soon as it becomes available. 一有货我们就会给你寄一本去。

(6) result in：造成；导致。

The cyclone has resulted in many thousands of deaths. 气旋已经造成了成千上万的人死亡。

(7) at (high) risk of sth: in：高风险。

(8) get rid of：摆脱；扔掉。

We get rid of all the old furniture. 我们扔掉了所有的旧家具。

(9) keep from：阻止；保护免受。

His only thought was to keep the boy from harm. 他一心想的就是不要让这男孩受到伤害。

COLD SYMPTOMS

COUGH　　HEADACHE　　HEAT　　COLD　　A SORE THROAT

Section C

Ⅰ Enhanced Learning【深度学习 自我预防】

1. Help Your Child Be a Germ Stopper

How Germs Spread

People who have the flu usually cough, sneeze, and have a runny nose. This makes droplets with virus in them. Other people can get the flu by breathing in these droplets or getting them in their nose or mouth. You can also get the flu by touching a hard surface such as a desk, doorknob, phone, or toy that has germs on it from a cough or sneeze and then touching your eyes, mouth, or nose before you wash your hands. We know that some viruses and bacteria (germs) can live for 2 or more hours on these hard surfaces.

What can you do to stop the spread of germs?

Take these 3 simple steps today!

Step 1—Cover your mouth and nose when you cough or sneeze. Teach your children to do the same.

How? Cough or sneeze into a tissue and then throw it away.

No tissue? Cough or sneeze into:

· Your sleeve (elbow) or shirt (shoulder).

Step 2—Clean your hands often. Teach your children to do the same

Wash your hands with soap and warm water. Do it for 20 seconds.

How long is 20 seconds?

· Count slowly to 20. Or wash long enough to sing the *Happy Handwashing Song* twice.

No soap around?

· Use hand gel or hand wipes.

Step 3—Remind your children to use good hygiene.

Follow up with your children to make sure they follow the rules of good hygiene:

· Set a good example.

· Praise children when they practice these ways to stop germs in their tracks.

2. 5 Steps to Good Hand Washing

Do you know the right way to wash your hands? Take these 5 simple steps to good hygiene.

Step 1—Turn on the warm water and let it run.

Turn on the warm water. If you have 2 faucets, turn on the cold first and then the hot until the water is warm.

Step 2—Wet your hands and soap up.

Get your hands wet by quickly running both hands under the warm water.

Turn one palm up flat under the soap nozzle and pump out some soap with your other hand. Or wet the bar of soap. Then rub the soap between your palms to make bubbles.

Rub your palms, the back of your hands, in between your fingers, and under your nails. Quickly dip your hands under the running water to make more bubbles and suds.

Step 3—Sing while you wash!

Lather up for at least 20 seconds. Sing the "Happy Hand Washing" song twice, the alphabet song. The 20 seconds will seem to fly by!

Step 4—Rinse off your hands.

Point your hands down into the sink so that the soap runs from your wrists to your fingertips. Make sure all the soap comes off.

Step 5—Dry off your hands.

Grab the paper towel and dry your hands. Then use the paper towel to turn off the faucet, and throw the paper away. At home, you can use a cloth towel and use bare hands to turn off the faucet.

Ⅱ Extensive Learning【拓展学习　媒体动态】

More than 3,700 Americans have tested positive for the novel coronavirus and at least 69 have died, according to data compiled by Johns Hopkins University and CBS News.

However, U.S. health officials say a relatively small percentage of children have tested positive for COVID-19 and those who have it tend to show milder symptoms. No child deaths have yet been reported.

By comparison, 36 million Americans have gotten the flu this season and about 22,000 have died. Children have been more vulnerable than years past with 144 pediatric deaths reported, according to the latest statistics from the CDC. Eight more child deaths were reported this week.

The figures underline a recent trend—while COVID-19 has largely spared children since its December outbreak in China, the flu has proven particularly devastating for kids in America this season. (In older people, however, coronavirus is much deadlier than the flu.)

Read more from
CBS News, 2020

Read more 4-1

The best way to protect yourself and your loved ones against influenza (flu) is to get a flu vaccine every flu season. Flu is a contagious respiratory disease that can lead to serious illness, hospitalization, or even death. CDC recommends everyone six months and older get an annual flu vaccine.

Flu vaccines have a good safety record. Hundreds of millions of Americans have safely received flu vaccines over the past 50 years. Extensive research supports the safety of seasonal flu vaccines. Each year, CDC works with the U.S. Food and Drug Administration (FDA) and other partners to ensure the highest safety standards for flu vaccines.

You should get a flu vaccine by the end of October. However, as long as flu viruses are circulating, vaccination should continue throughout flu season, even in January or later.

Read more from
CDC, 2018

Read more 4-2

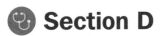 Section D

Practice【实践探索　行动项目】

Key 4-2

1. Project 1

Hand Washing Word Scramble

Unscramble the words below. See if you can do this handout without using the hints.

		Hint:	Answer:
(1)	mgser	These are what make you sick.	_____
(2)	svuri	This is one type of germ.	_____
(3)	dsnha	What you should always wash.	_____
(4)	gnnirun trwae	What you wash your hands with.	_____
(5)	diquli sapo	Helps to get rid of germs.	_____
(6)	seaidse	What germs can cause.	_____
(7)	cibaceatr	This is another type of germ.	_____
(8)	lehahyt	Washing your hands can keep you	_____

2. Project 2

Lesson plan & practice: Suggest you are a teacher in a kindergarten or a childcare center, you are trying to teach the children about flu and handwashing. Try to make with your group members a "Hand Washing Lesson Plan" for children ages 3 to 7 and practice your lesson plan in the class.

Key 4-3

Section E

Self-assessment【进阶评估　自我超越】

1. Cooperative Learning Assessment

Please check your contribution to the group after the project is done.

	Superior (5)	Above Average (4)	Average (3)	Below Average (2)	Weak (1)
Understood what was required for the project					
Participated in the group discussion					
Helped the group to function well as a team					
Contributed useful ideas					
How much work was done					
Quality of completed work					
What could you improve upon next time?					
Your group members' comments					
Your group leader's comments					

2. Assessment of Your Study

Instructions:

(1) Read each statement in the table below and place a check mark in the column that best describes how well you can complete that task.

(2) Review your responses for each task. If you have checked five or more in the "Somewhat" and / or "No" columns, you may need to consider making greater efforts after class.

I can	Yes	Somewhat	No
Understand the main idea of the text			
Identify the major points, important facts and details, and vocabulary in the text			
Make inferences about what is implied in the text			
Recognize the organization and purpose of the text			
Remember the new words and expressions			
Speak on the topic effectively			
Employ search strategy to gain information to address the project			
Refer to appropriate resources to deal with the project			

3. Personal Development

Instruction:

Completing this section will help you make informed practicing decisions. Please identify your strengths and the areas that you need to develop or strengthen and record them below.

STRENGTHS:
I am confident that I can...
(1)
(2)
(3)
AREAS FOR IMPROVEMENT:
I would like to improve my ability to...
(1)
(2)
(3)

4. Say What You Want to Say

Please start what you want to say.

Unit 2　Baby Teeth Care
牙齿护理

Section A

Warm-up Activity【听歌记词　护牙卫生】

Video 4-2

1. **Listen to the Kids' Song *Brush Your Teeth* and Try to Get the Lyrics（Video 4-2）**

_____

_____

_____

_____

_____

2. **Do's and Don'ts for Dental Health**

Brush your tooth every day (　　)

Smoke tobacco (　　)

Drink water, black & green tea (　　)

Crunch on ice (　　)

See your dentist regularly (　　)

Sleeping disorder (　　)

Eat a lot of sweet things (　　)

Eat fiber-filled vegetables and fruits (　　)

Section B

Ⅰ Picture Book【绘本阅读　牙齿趣识】

Tooth Fairy

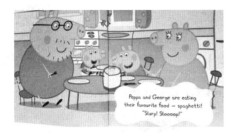

Peppa and George are eating their favorite food-spaghetti (意大利面)!

"Slurp (吃东西时发出啧啧的声音)! Sloooop!"

Suddenly something falls on to Peppa's plate.

"What's that?" Peppa cries.

"It's your tooth!" Daddy Pig laughs.

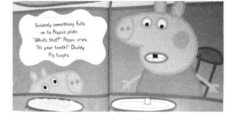

"If you put the tooth under your pillow (枕头) tonight the Tooth Fairy will pay you a visit.

She will take the tooth and leave you a shiny coin!" says Mummy Pig.

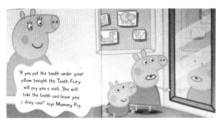

"Goodnight, Peppa! Goodnight, George!"says Mummy Pig.

"Goodnight, my little piggies!" grunts (咕哝) Daddy Pig.

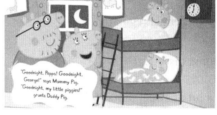

Peppa puts her tooth under the pillow for the Tooth Fairy.

"Let's stay awake all night and see the Tooth Fairy." says Peppa.

"Snort!" George giggles (咯咯地笑).

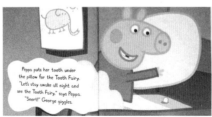

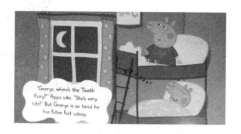

"George, where's the Tooth Fairy?" Peppa asks.

"She's very late!"

But George is so tired he has fallen fast asleep.

"I'm not going to go... to... sleep... I'm... zzzzzz," snores (打呼噜) Peppa.

When everything is quiet, something appears at the window.

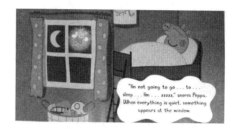

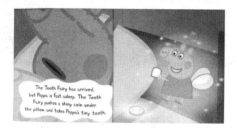

The Tooth Fairy has arrived, but Peppa is fast asleep.

The Tooth Fairy pushes a shiny coin under the pillow

and takes Peppa's tiny tooth.

Peppa, George, wake up! It's morning." says Mummy Pig brightly.

"Did the Tooth Fairy come?" Daddy Pig asks.

"No." says Peppa sadly.

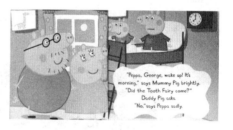

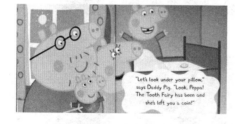

"Let's look under your pillow." says Daddy Pig.

"Look, Peppa! "

The Tooth Fairy has been and she's left you a coin!"

Hooray! Hee! Hee! Hee!" Peppa laughs.

"Grunt! Next time I will stay awake and I will see the Tooth Fairy! Hee! Hee!"

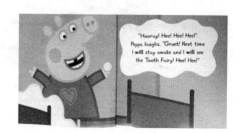

Ⅱ Notes【说文解字　名词注释】

1. Vocabulary Table

Vocabulary 4-2

Words & Expressions	Part of Speech	Meaning in Text
spaghetti	*n.*	意大利面
slurp	*v.*	啧啧吃的声音
pillow	*n.*	枕头
grunt	*n.*	咕哝着说
giggle	*n.*	咯咯地笑
snore	*v.*	打呼噜

2. Useful Knowledge

(1) tooth fairy：牙仙子。

牙仙子是西方国家和西方文化中的一位精灵,最早起源于北欧,叫作tand-fé,相传小孩睡觉时,把掉下来的乳牙放到枕头下面,牙仙子就会降临把牙齿取走,并根据牙齿的优劣留下相应价值的一点零花钱作为回报。这个传统在很多西方国家盛行,让很多孩子的换牙阶段变成了备受期待的妙趣旅程。

Resource 4-2

(2) spaghetti：意大利面。

spaghetti是意大利面的其中一种,英语中的意大利面的统称叫作pasta,常见的有以下几种:

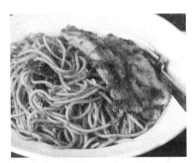
Spaghetti 意大利式细面条

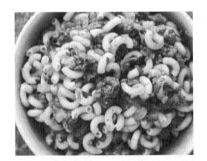
Macaroni 通心粉

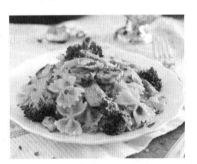
Farfalle 蝴蝶面

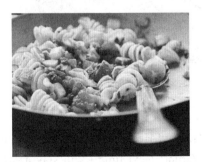
Fusilli 意大利螺旋面

(3) leave 在文中表示留下、剩下。

Your shoes left muddy marks on the floor. 地板上都是你鞋底留的泥印子。

leave 还可以表示使保留；使保持某种状态。

Leave me alone. 让我一个人待着／不要打扰我。

leave 还可以表示离开、离去。需要注意的是，想表达从某地离开时，leave 后面直接加地点，不需要接介词 from。

He left the house by the back door. 他从房子的后门离开了。

(4) milk tooth：乳牙。

(5) pay a visit (to visit a person or place)：拜访；参观。

eg: If you have time, pay a visit to the City Art Gallery. 如果你有时间，可以去参观城市美术馆。

(6) stay awake (keep not sleeping)：保持清醒。

eg: He finds it so difficult to stay awake during history lessons. 他觉得上历史课不打瞌睡太难了。

(7) fast asleep (sleeping deeply)：熟睡。

eg: Going upstairs five minutes later, she was fast asleep. 上楼五分钟后她就睡熟了。

Section C

Ⅰ Enhanced Learning【深度学习　牙齿卫士】

Get to know the names of milk and permanent teeth with the following two pictures, and try to finish the following table about baby teeth development.

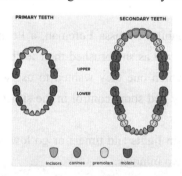
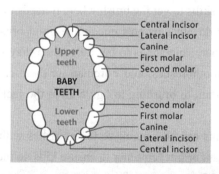

	Name	Name (Chinese)	Age Tooth Comes In	Age Tooth Falls Out
Upper Teeth	central incisor			
	lateral incisor			
	canine			
	first molar			
	second molar			
Lower Teeth	central incisor			
	lateral incisor			
	canine			
	first molar			
	second molar			

Ⅱ Extensive Learning【拓展学习　媒体动态】

The Most Common Dental Health Issues in Kids

Having healthy pearly whites is as important for children as it is for adults. Following are some suggestions from pediatric dentists on how to avoid common kids' dental health problems. Here's to a healthy smile for a lifetime!

Visit the Dentist Regularly—And Early

It probably comes as no surprise that cavities top the list of dental issues among patients ages 1 to 18, according to Dr. Robert Delarosa, DDS, a pediatric dentist in Baton Rouge, La., and the president-elect of the American Academy of Pediatric Dentistry. Although cavities can cause a lot of problems, most of the time, they're preventable.

The first line of defense is regular dental visits. Six months is the standard time between visits, but children who are more at risk for cavities—some patients with special needs or children who have a family history of tooth decay or who wear orthodontic appliances, for example—may require more frequent trips.

Brush to Keep Decay Away

Parents need to take children's brushing and flossing into their own hands to ensure good results. The AAPD recommends children (and grown-ups) brush for two minutes twice a day and floss at least once a day. Though toddlers and preschoolers are all about doing tasks independently, dental care should not be one of those things, say both Moody and Delarosa. "For a young child, you're going to have to brush and floss for them," says Moody. "They're not capable of doing a really good job by themselves until about age 7 or 8. They just don't yet have the motor skills to get the brush where it needs to go."

How do other parents encourage good brushing habits? Melissa Foreman, a Pennsylvania mom of four, sang songs to her kids when they were young as she brushed their teeth. Each kid had two toothbrushes, and Foreman let them choose which one they wanted to use when they were resistant to brushing to "give them the feeling they had some control in the situation," she says.

Parents can also purchase toothbrushes with built-in lights and timers or go low-tech with an hourglass or kitchen timer to ensure kids do the full two minutes.

Diet Matters

Certainly a steady diet of Skittles and soda will create a breeding ground for cavities, but parents should be mindful of all refined carbohydrates their children consume, including kiddo faves like juice, crackers and baked treats. "Things that have a high sugar content and are high refined carbohydrates that can stay on the tooth structure, those are problems for us," says Delarosa.

Sodas and juices pack a double whammy of sugar and acid, making the teeth extra-vulnerable, but even diet versions of the drinks are highly acidic and bad for teeth enamel. When kids are thirsty, Delarosa says, give them water. The AAPD recommends kids drink no more than 4 to 6 ounces of juice a day, preferably with breakfast and followed by brushing. (Likewise, the American Academy of Pediatrics recommends 4 to 6 ounces of juice per day for kids ages 1 to 6, and 8 to 12 ounces for kids ages 7 to 18.)

Kids, especially toddlers and teenagers, tend to be "grazers," says Delarosa, meaning they often consume snacks and sugary drinks all day long. He recommends parents establish regular snack and meal times to cut down on all-day munching and curb the constant contact of sugar on the teeth. Avoid sending little kids to bed with bottles or sippy cups of milk or juice.

☆For your reference

To get to know more information about child teeth care, you may visit:

(1) http://www.mychildrensteeth.org/.

(The American Academy of Pediatric Dentistry)

(2) https://supersimple.com/?s = teeth.

(songs & videos)

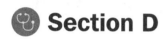 # Section D

Projects in Practice【实践探索　行动项目】

1. Project 1

Presentation: 演讲展示

Share the teeth culture and customs in your hometown, you may talk about how people dispose baby's falling tooth and why.

2. Project 2

Role Play: 角色扮演

Try to act out the *Tooth Fairy* story in Section B with your partners.（Video 4–3）

Video 4–3

Section E

Self-assessment【进阶评估　自我超越】

1. Cooperative Learning Assessment

Please check your contribution to the group after the project is done.

	Superior (5)	Above Average (4)	Average (3)	Below Average (2)	Weak (1)
Understood what was required for the project					
Participated in the group discussion					
Helped the group to function well as a team					
Contributed useful ideas					
How much work was done					
Quality of completed work					
What could you improve upon next time?					
Your group members' comments					
Your group leader's comments					

2. Assessment of Your Study

Instructions:

(1) Read each statement in the table below and place a check mark in the column that best describes how well you can complete that task.

(2) Review your responses for each task. If you have checked five or more in the "Somewhat" and / or "No" columns, you may need to consider making greater efforts after class.

I can	Yes	Somewhat	No
Understand the main idea of the text			
Identify the major points, important facts and details, and vocabulary in the text			
Make inferences about what is implied in the text			
Recognize the organization and purpose of the text			
Remember the new words and expressions			
Speak on the topic effectively			
Employ search strategy to gain information to address the project			
Refer to appropriate resources to deal with the project			

3. Personal Development

Instruction:

Completing this section will help you make informed practicing decisions. Please identify your strengths and the areas that you need to develop or strengthen and record them below.

STRENGTHS:
I am confident that I can...
(1)
(2)
(3)
AREAS FOR IMPROVEMENT:
I would like to improve my ability to...
(1)
(2)
(3)

4. Say What You Want to Say

Please start what you want to say.

Unit 3　Baby Massage
婴儿抚触

🩺 Section A

Warm-up Activity【宝宝抚触　健康关爱】

Here are some preparations for baby massage. Please tick the right answers based upon the video "Introduction to BaBy Massage"（Video 4-4）.

Pillow (　　)　　　　Towel (　　)　　　　Swaddle (　　)

Sunflower oil (　　)　　Olive oil (　　)　　　Coconut oil (　　)

Nut oils (　　)　　　　Complex ingredients oils (　　)

Video 4-4

🩺 Section B

Key 4-4

Ⅰ　Know About Baby Massage【婴儿照护　温暖抚触】

What Is Baby Massage?

Baby massage is a longstanding (长久的) parenting (养育) tradition in many cultures, including Indian and African, and was introduced to the western world during the last 30 years, gaining in popularity in the U.K. since the late 1990's.

Baby massage is when a parent or primary carer (护理员) lovingly strokes (轻抚) or holds their baby. Using a high quality non-fragrance (非香料) vegetable oil, soothing holds and rhythmic strokes are given on each area of baby's body, following a sequence (先后次序) that has been developed over many years. The massage offers a wonderful experience and a special time to communicate both verbally and non-verbally with babies, so that they feel loved, valued and respected.

The Benefits of Baby Massage

The benefits of baby massage can be divided into four categories: stimulation; relaxation; relief; and interaction. The four main sources for baby massage strokes are developed from Indian and Swedish massage, foot massage using reflexology (反射论) techniques, and strokes and combinations drawn from Yoga.

As the parent gains confidence, their self-esteem is enhanced and the benefits to the parent and infant are enormous (巨大的). The parent should gain good inter-personal skills and confidence in a social situation. The skills gained from this experience are life long and can be passed down the family networks. By being stroked, and caressed (爱抚),and carried, and cuddled (拥抱),

comforted, and cooed (柔声地说) to, by being loved, the child learns to love others . Feeling loved and valued and supported by a network of reliable affectionate (充满深情的) relationships is going to enhance the parent and baby mental well-being (健康).

Getting Started of Baby Massage

Before you get started, make sure you're in a quiet, calming environment, you're using a soft surface (操作台), and you have some good-quality baby cream or massage oil. Make sure you use a cream or oil gentle enough for your baby's sensitive skin.

Timing is key here. Don't try to massage your baby just before or after a meal, or when she's tired or needs a nap. You can choose to remove all your baby's clothes if the room is warm enough, or keep on the diaper (尿布), just in case.

Place your baby on a soft, warm towel on the bed or on the floor. Remove any jewelry that may catch, rub (擦), or irritate (刺激) your baby's skin. Always rub the cream or oil in your hands before making contact with your baby to warm both your hands and the cream. Your hands may soak up (吸收) the first lot (批). Just add some more; your hands obviously need it too.

Watch your baby's reaction to each movement, and if she doesn't like anything, stop what you're doing and give your baby a cuddle instead.

Ⅱ Notes【说文解字　名词注释】

1. Vocabulary Table

Vocabulary 4-3

Words & Expressions	Part of Speech	Meaning in Text
longstanding	*adj.*	长时间的;长期存在的
parenting	*n.*	养育;抚养;教养
carer	*n.*	看护者;照料者
stroke	*vt.*	轻抚;抚摸
non-fragranced	*adj.*	无香味的;非香料
sequence	*n.*	有关联的一组事物;先后次序
reflexology	*n.*	反射论
enormous	*adj.*	巨大的;极大的
caress	*vt.*	爱抚;抚摸
cuddle	*vt.&n.*	拥抱;怀抱
coo	*vi*	柔声地说
affectionate	*adj.*	充满深情的;温柔亲切的
well-being	*n.*	健康;幸福
surface	*n.*	操作台
diaper	*n.*	尿布
rub	*vt.*	擦;磨;搓
irritate	*vt.*	刺激(皮肤或身体部位)
soak up	phr.	吸收
lot	n.	份;组

2. Useful Knowledge

(1) Yoga is a group of physical, mental, and spiritual practices or disciplines which originated in ancient India. There is a broad variety of yoga schools, practices, and goals in Hinduism, Buddhism, and Jainism. Among the most well-known types of yoga are Hatha yoga and Rāja yoga.

(2) Sensitive skin is a skin condition in which skin is prone to itching and irritation experienced as a subjective sensation when using cosmetics and toiletries. When questioned, over 50% of women in the UK and US, and 38% of men, report that they have sensitive skin.

(3) A diaper (American English) or a nappy (British English) is a type of underwear that allows the wearer to defecate or urinate without the use of a toilet, by absorbing or containing waste products to prevent soiling of outer clothing or the external environment. When diapers become soiled, they require changing, generally by a second person such as a parent or caregiver. Failure to change a diaper on a sufficiently regular basis can result in skin problems around the area covered by the diaper.

Diapers are made of cloth or synthetic disposable materials. Cloth diapers are composed of layers of fabric such as cotton, hemp, bamboo, microfiber, or even plastic fibers such as PLA, and can be washed and reused multiple times. Disposable diapers contain absorbent chemicals and are thrown away after use. Plastic pants can be worn over diapers to avoid leaks, but with modern cloth diapers, this is no longer necessary.

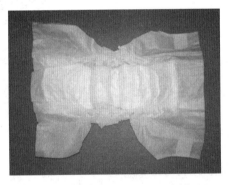

Disposable baby diaper with resealable tapes and elasticated leg cuffs

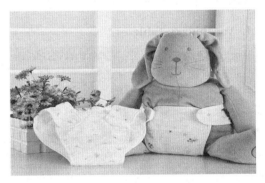

Outer diapers

Section C

Ⅰ Enhanced Learning【深度学习　实景训练】

How to Massage Your Baby

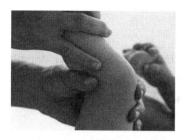

The Legs

Her legs are a good place to begin, as they're less sensitive than some parts of her body. Using a little oil, wrap your hands around one of her thighs and pull down, one hand after the other, squeezing gently, as if you're "milking" her leg. Switch legs and repeat.

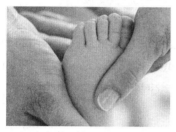

The Feet

Take one foot and gently rotate it a few times in each direction, then stroke the top of her foot from the ankle down to the toes. Switch feet and repeat.

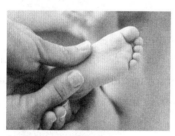

The Soles

Use your thumbs to trace circles all over the bottom of each foot.

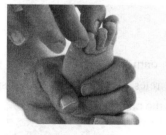

The Toes

To finish off the feet, take each toe between your thumb and forefinger and gently pull until your fingers slip off the end. Repeat for all ten toes.

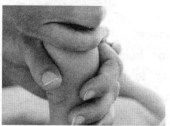

The Arms

Take one of her arms in your hands and repeat the milking motion from her armpit all the way to her wrist. Then, take her hand and gently rotate her wrist a few times in each direction. Switch arms and repeat.

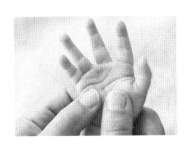

The Hands

Trace tiny circles over the palm of each of her hands with your thumbs.

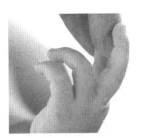

The Fingers

Gently take a finger between your thumb and forefinger and pull, letting her finger slip through your grasp. Repeat for all her fingers and both thumbs.

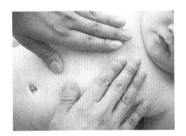

The Chest

Place your hands together in prayer position over her heart. Then, opening out your hands slowly, stroke outward and lightly flatten the palms over her chest. Repeat several times.

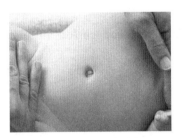

The Chest (continued)

Place one hand flat across the top of her chest. Stroke it gently down to her thighs. Repeat the motion, alternating hands, several times.

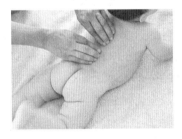

The Back

Roll your baby onto her tummy. Using your fingertips, trace tiny circles on either side of her spine from the neck down to the buttocks.

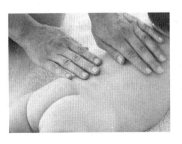

The Back (continued)

Finish with some long, firm strokes from her shoulders all the way to her feet. When you have finished, put on her nappy and cuddle or breastfeed her. She'll probably doze off!

Ⅱ Extensive Learning【拓展学习　媒体动态】

Should I use oil to massage my baby?

Using an oil can make massage easier for you and more relaxing for your baby.

Everyone seems to have an opinion on which oil is best for baby massage. Some parents favour baby mineral oils, while others choose a particular vegetable oil. Some oils are thought to be more easily absorbed into skin. You may find massage easier with an oil that soaks in, or you may prefer one that stays more slippery on your baby's skin.

Your decision about what to use also depends on your baby's skin. If your baby has eczema, it is better to use her medical emollient cream or ointment.

There are some oils or creams that it's best not to use, whether or not your baby has eczema.

Read more from
Indian Pediatr , 2010

Read more 4-3

Massage may help your baby to sleep as part of her bedtime routine.

Research suggests that massaging your baby regularly may help to get her circadian rhythms on track, meaning she'll sleep more at night and be more active during the day.

Your baby's circadian rhythm influences the physical and mental changes that her body goes through every 24 hours or so. The natural rise and fall of your baby's appetite, body temperature, and her readiness for sleep, all reflect her circadian rhythm.

Our bodies usually prepare for sleep when it gets dark. When the day's light fades, our brain responds by producing the hormone melatonin.

Melatonin helps to slow us down and make us drowsy. It continues to be released throughout our sleep at night. The more we sleep during the dark night hours, the more melatonin our brains will produce.

Read more from
Baby Centre, 2020.

Read more 4-4

A regular massage is a great way to help dads and their babies to feel closer. Your partner could make massage part of your baby's bedtime routine.

Dads who massage their babies do tend to have a closer relationship with them. These dads often get more involved in other areas of babycare too, such as bathtime and floor play.

It works both ways. Babies who are massaged by their dads are more connected to their dads. If babies have enjoyed this close physical contact with their dads, they get more excited when they see their dads. They smile, reach for, and call out to their dads more readily than babies who haven't been massaged.

If your partner is reluctant to try massage, it may be because he's never thought of it as something he would do as a dad. He may need time to get used to the idea. Ask your health visitor if there are baby massage classes in your area. There may even be classes just for dads.

Read more from
Baby Center, 2017

Read more 4-5

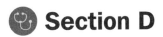 Section D

Projects in Practice【实践探索　挑战自我】

1. Project 1

Follow the step-by-step guide based on the video "Baby Massage" (Video 4-5) to learn the techniques for massaging a baby.

Video 4-5

2. Project 2

Situational Play

Suggest you are a teacher in a childcare center, and you are trying to teach parents about baby massage. Try to act out with your group members.

Possible discussion topics:

(1) Whether massage is good to my baby?

(2) How to massage my baby?

(3) How to choose oils for baby massage?

Section E

Self-assessment【进阶评估　自我超越】

1. Cooperative Learning Assessment

Please check your contribution to the group after the project is done.

	Superior (5)	Above Average (4)	Average (3)	Below Average (2)	Weak (1)
Understood what was required for the project					
Participated in the group discussion					
Helped the group to function well as a team					
Contributed useful ideas					
How much work was done					
Quality of completed work					
What could you improve upon next time?					
Your group members' comments					
Your group leader's comments					

2. Assessment of Individual Study

Instructions:

(1) Read each statement in the table below and place a check mark in the column that best describes how well you can complete that task.

(2) Review your responses for each task. If you have checked five or more in the "Somewhat" and / or "No" columns, you may need to consider making greater efforts after class.

I can	Yes	Somewhat	No
Understand the main idea of the text			
Identify the major points, important facts and details, and vocabulary in the text			
Make inferences about what is implied in the text			
Recognize the organization and purpose of the text			
Remember the new words and expressions			
Speak on the topic effectively			
Employ search strategy to gain information to address the project			
Refer to appropriate resources to deal with the project			

3. Personal Development

Instruction:

Completing this section will help you make informed practicing decisions. Please identify your strengths and the areas that you need to develop or strengthen and record them below.

STRENGTHS:
I am confident that I can...

(1)

(2)

(3)

AREAS FOR IMPROVEMENT:
I would like to improve my ability to...

(1)

(2)

(3)

Chapter 5

Elderly Care

夕阳有约

Unit 1　The Art of Care

照护艺术

Section A

Warm-up Activity【远离疾病　守护健康】

Video 5–1

1. Let's Keep the Following Sign Language in Our Mind

A	B	C

D	E

(1) _____ (2) _____ (3) _____ (4) _____ (5) _____

2. Let's Listen and Repeat the Sentence You Hear by Yourself

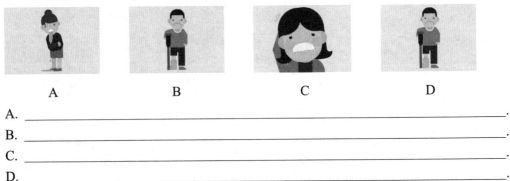

A　　　　　　　B　　　　　　　C　　　　　　　D

A. _____.
B. _____.
C. _____.
D. _____.

Section B

Key 5-1

I Passage:The Art of Care【用心守护　照护艺术】

Care is a work of labor (劳动) and toil (辛勤劳作) with mind and body. Preparation of meal, feeding, assistance (协助) in displacement, assistance in bathing, accompanying the cared-for to visit a physician, communication with the patient/ward, and interaction (相互交流) with other family members of the patient are all parts of the care work. A caregiver is sometimes in a state of nervousness and confusion (迷茫), most of the time afraid that there might be a possible mistake.

As caregivers (家庭护理员), we must have "patience", "perseverance" (毅力) and "concentration" as well as "kindness" and "sincerity" (真诚) towards these works. During the process of taking care of the patients or wards (病房病人), this will agitate a different spark. Therefore, "caretaking is also an art."

Nevertheless, in order to make yourself more proficient in caretaking and to accomplish (完成) the work with ease, you need to fully learn certain diseases and all kinds of care knowledge and skills.

Furthermore, apart from (除了……以外还有) busy taking care of the patient or ward, caregivers also have to pay attention to their own physical and mental state at all times. Once you have a physical or mental discomfort (不舒服), you should let the employer know and avoid (避免) bearing the burden alone. It is important and necessary to learn self protection.

The work of care is tedious (冗长的) and painstaking (需细心的). However, it is also an important process for mutual support and care among people. It is an act of love. Because of you, families and the society become more stable (稳定的) and wonderful.

(*Source:* Taipei City Foreign Caregivers Manual, 2014)

II Notes【说文解字　名词注释】

1. Vocabulary Table

Vocabulary 5-1

Words & Expressions	Part of Speech	Meaning in Text
labor	*n.*	劳动;努力
toil	*n.*	(长时间)苦干;辛勤劳作
assistance	*n.*	帮助;援助;支持
interaction	*n.*	相互影响(作用,制约)
confusion	*n.*	不确定;困惑;混淆
caregiver	*n.*	照料家居老弱病患者的人;家庭护理员
perseverance	*n.*	毅力;韧性;不屈不挠的精神
sincerity	*n.*	诚意;真挚
ward	*n.*	病房;病室

Words & Expressions	Part of Speech	Meaning in Text
accomplish	*vt.*	完成
apart from	*phr.*	除了……外(都)
discomfort	*n.*	轻微的病痛;不舒服;不适
avoid	*vt.*	避免;防止
tedious	*adj.*	冗长的;啰唆的;单调乏味的
painstaking	*adj.*	需细心的;辛苦的;需专注的
stable	*adj.*	稳定的;稳固的;牢固的

2. Read Following Me

(1) How to read a passage?

Key 5-2

Step 1　Find the key sentence of each paragraph.

Step 2　Divide the passage into 3 parts.

Step 3　Write down the main idea of each part.

Step 4　Answer the following questions.

Q1. Why we say "caretaking is an art"?

_____ .

Q2: What should caregivers have during their work?

_____ .

Q3: Why should caregivers pay attention to their own health condition?

_____ .

Q4: What is the key point of the "art" of care according to the passage?

_____ .

Q5: Why do we need caregivers?

_____ .

(2) How to read a sentence?

① It is an act of love.

Step 1　It is an act.

这是一种艺术。

Step 2　It is an act *of love*.

这是一种爱的艺术。

② Care is a work of labor and toil with mind and body.

Step 1　Care is a work.

照护是一份工作。

Step 2　Care is a work *of labor and toil*.

照护是一份辛苦劳动的工作。

Step 3　Care is a work *of labor and toil with mind and body*.

照护是一份既劳心又劳力的工作。

③ Preparation of meal, feeding, assistance in displacement, assistance in bathing, accompanying the cared-for to visit a physician, communication with the patient / ward, and interaction with other family members of the patient are all parts of the care work.

Step 1　Preparation, feeding, assistance, assistance, accompanying, communication, and interaction are all care work.

准备、喂食、协助、协助、陪伴、交流和互动都是照护工作。

Step 2　Preparation *of meal*, feeding, assistance *in displacement*, assistance *in bathing*, accompanying sb. to do sth, communication *with the patient / ward*, and interaction *with other family members* of the patient are all *parts of* the care work.

备餐、喂食、协助移位、协助淋浴、陪伴某人、与被爱护人沟通、与其他家庭成员互动都是照护工作的一部分。

Step 3　Preparation of meal, feeding, assistance in displacement, assistance in bathing, accompanying *the cared-for* to *visit a physician*, communication with the patient / ward, and interaction with other family members *of the patient* are all parts of the care work.

备餐、喂食、协助移位、协助淋浴、陪伴就医、与被爱护人沟通、与被爱护人的其他家庭成员互动都是照护工作的一部分。

(3) How to read words and expressions?

Step 1　About the care work.

Labor and toil; tedious and painstaking; an act of love.

Preparation of meal, feeding, assistance in displacement, assistance in bathing, accompany the cared-for to visit a physician, communication with the patient / ward, interaction with family members.

Step 2　About caregivers.

Patience, perseverance, concentration, kindness, sincerity, nervousness and confusion, proficient.

Step 3　About the society.

Stable and wonderful.

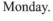 # Section C

I Extensive Learning【深度学习　优质照护】

Aging China Needs Professional Elderly Care

The shortage of nursing staff (员工) has been a bottleneck (瓶颈) for China's elderly care services and the aging society calls for more professional employees, said China Youth Daily Monday.

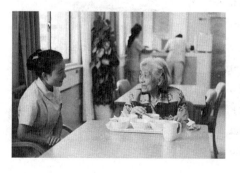

With nearly 41 million disabled or semi-disabled (半残疾的) senior citizens, the country should have at least 13 million elderly nursing staff according to international standards. However, there were less than half a million elderly care professionals in 2017, with only 20,000 of them certified (有专业证书), said the newspaper citing a report from Beijing Normal

University (BNU).

The lack of colleges which offer elderly care as a major, along with inadequate (不足) social acceptance (接受认同) and low salary around 4,000 to 5,000 yuan ($579 to $724) fail to cultivate (培养) and attract more people going into this field, said the newspaper.

Over two-thirds of college students studying elderly care come from rural families and more than 70 percent of the students expect monthly incomes between 3,001 to 7,000 yuan, according to an employment report released by the China Philanthropy (慈善事业) Research Institute at BNU.

The report found positive changes in elderly care, said Cheng Feifei, director of the institute, adding that at least half of the surveyed (调研) families were neutral (中立的) or supportive of elderly care services.

The institute called for more subsidies (补贴) for elderly care students as well as more cooperation between schools and employers to facilitate (促进) the employment of students.

At the end of 2018, China had a population of 249 million aged 60 or above, and the number is expected to exceed (超过) 300 million in 2025, according to the National Health Commission.

(*Source: China Daily*, 3 June 2019)

Ⅱ Extensive Learning【拓展学习　岗位应用】

1. How to Measure Blood Pressure（Video5-2）

Preparation for Necessary Items 用物准备：

An electronic sphygmomanometer, a record book, a pen

电子血压计、记录本、笔

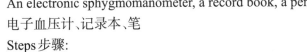

Video 5-2

Steps 步骤：

(1) Assist the patient or ward to take a comfortable sitting or lying position. A small pillow, small bath towel or bed sheet can be used to support the arm. 协助被看护人采用舒适的坐姿或卧姿，手臂可用小枕头、小浴巾或被单支托。

(2) Roll up the sleeve of the arm of the patient or ward to the upper arm or pull the sleeve straight, then find the position of the brachial artery and make sure that the brachial artery position is at the same level as the heart. 将被看护人一宿卷至上臂或将袖子拉平顺，找出肱动脉位置，使肱动脉位置与心脏同高。

(3) Place the blood pressure monitor in a smooth place, and have the palm of the patient facing up; wrap the cuff around the upper arm, and lower edge of the cuff should be 2-3 cm away from the cubital fossa. You should be able to insert 2 straight fingers between the cuff and the arm for an accurate fit. If there is a mark " ♂ " (midpoint of force application of the inflatable bag) on the cuff, then you should let the mark aim at the

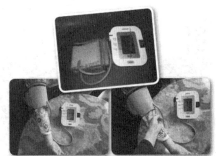

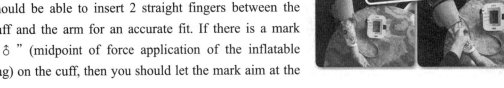

brachial artery. 血压计放平平稳之处，让被看护人手心朝上，将压脉带缠绕在上臂，压脉带下缘位置须距肘关节窝2—3cm处。压脉带松紧以深入两平指为宜，若压带上有"ծ"记号 (充气囊之施力中点)，则将之对准肱动脉。

(4) Press the measuring button. 按下测量键。

(5) Make sure you have a correct reading, and then remove the cuff. 确定测量结果，取下压脉带。

(6) Record the measured data, such as: 120 / 80 mmHg. 记录数据，例如：120 / 80 mmHg。

(*Source:* Taipei City Foreign Caregivers Manual, 2014)

2. Blood Pressure Assessment

Nurse: Hello, Mr. Johnson. Can I please check your blood pressure? 您好，约翰逊先生，我可以给您量血压吗？

Patient: Sure. 好。

Nurse: Can you roll up your sleeves? 您可以卷起袖子吗？

Patient: Of course. 好的。

Nurse: I'm going to check your blood pressure now. 我现在开始测了。

Patient: Is it OK? 我的血压还好吗？

Nurse: It is a little high today. 今天有点高。

Patient: Oh... What's my blood pressure today? 哦。我今天的血压多少？

Nurse: It's 160 / 95. It's higher than usual. Did you take your blood pressure medication this morning? 您的血压是160 / 95，有一点高。您今天吃高血压的药了吗？

Patient: Oh no, I forgot to take it. 哎呀，没有，我忘记吃了。

Nurse: I will get it for your now. 我现在给您去拿药

Patient: Thanks! I should take it every morning. 谢谢！我一定要记得每天早晨吃。

(*Source:* Alanna Tu , 27 March 2019)

Notes

Before we take blood pressure of patients, we should make a simple assessment. 当我们在给患者测量血压之前，我们通常需要做一些简单的评估。

(1) Before I take/check your blood pressure, could you please tell me if you have had any previous surgeries done on either your chest or arms? 在我给您量血压之前，您可以告诉我您以前做过胸部或手臂的手术吗？

(2) Do you have any history of high blood pressure? 您有高血压吗？

(3) What is your blood pressure usually like? 您一般血压是多少？

(4) Have you had/taken any medication for your blood pressure today? 您今天有吃过高血压药吗？

3. High Blood Pressure

High blood pressure should be treated earlier with lifestyle changes and in some patients with medication (药物治疗) —at 130 / 80 mm Hg rather than 140 / 90—based on new ACC and American Heart Association (AHA) guidelines for the detection (侦查), prevention (预防),

management and treatment of high blood pressure.

High blood pressure (also referred to as HBP, or hypertension) is when your blood pressure, the force of blood flowing (流动) through your blood vessels, is consistently too high.

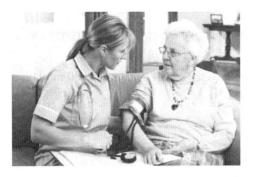

If you have high blood pressure, you are not alone. Nearly half of American adults have high blood pressure. (Many don't even know they have it.) The best way to know if you have high blood pressure, it is to have your blood pressure checked. Know your numbers. Learn about your blood pressure numbers and what they mean.

Blood Pressure Categories

BLOOD PRESSURE CATEGORY	SYSTOLIC mm Hg (upper number)		DIASTOLIC mm Hg (lower number)
NORMAL	LESS THAN 120	and	LESS THAN 80
ELEVATED	120 – 129	and	LESS THAN 80
HIGH BLOOD PRESSURE (HYPERTENSION) STAGE 1	130 – 139	or	80 – 89
HIGH BLOOD PRESSURE (HYPERTENSION) STAGE 2	140 OR HIGHER	or	90 OR HIGHER
HYPERTENSIVE CRISIS (consult your doctor immediately)	HIGHER THAN 180	and/or	HIGHER THAN 120

High blood pressure is a "silent killer". Most of the time there are no obvious symptoms (症状). Certain physical traits (特质) and lifestyle choices can put you at a greater risk for high blood pressure. When left untreated, the damage that high blood pressure does to your circulatory (循环) system is a significant (重要的) contributing factor to heart attack, stroke (打击) and other health threats.

(*Source:*American Heart Association National Center)

Section D

Projects in Practice【实践探索　行动项目】

1. Project 1

Make a dialogue: Practice blood pressure assessment with your classmates like caregivers and wards.

Caregiver: Hello, Mr. Johnson. May I please check your blood pressure? 您好,约翰逊先生,我可以给您量血压吗?

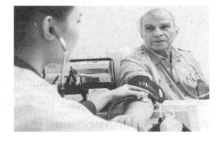

Ward: Sure. 好。

Caregiver: ...

Ward: ...

2. Project 2

Scene Play: Take blood pressure for some of your classmates, teachers, family members or friends and write theirs numbers down.

Name	Age	Record	Blood Pressure Category			Result
			Blood Pressure Category	Systolic (Upper #)	Diastolic (Lower #)	
Li li	39	108/64	Normal	Leaa than 120	Less than 80	Normal
			Prehypertansion	120—139	80—89	
			High Blood Pressure (Hypertension) Stage 1	140—159	90—99	
			High Blood Pressure (Hypertension) Stage 1	160 or Higher	100 or Higher	
			High Blood Pressure (Hypertension) Stage 1	Higher than 180	Higher than 110	

3. Project 3

Understand the blood pressure.（Video 5–3）

Video 5–3

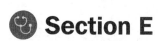 Section E

Self-assessment【进阶评估　自我超越】

1. About New Words and Phrases

How many new words and phrases have been committed in your memory? Please write them down.

（1）Care work:＿＿＿＿＿＿＿＿＿＿＿＿＿＿＿＿＿＿＿＿＿＿＿＿

＿＿＿＿＿＿＿＿＿＿＿＿＿＿＿＿＿＿＿＿＿＿＿＿＿＿＿＿＿＿＿＿＿＿

＿＿＿＿＿＿＿＿＿＿＿＿＿＿＿＿＿＿＿＿＿＿＿＿＿＿＿＿＿＿＿＿＿＿

（2）Blood pressure:＿＿＿＿＿＿＿＿＿＿＿＿＿＿＿＿＿＿＿＿＿＿＿

＿＿＿＿＿＿＿＿＿＿＿＿＿＿＿＿＿＿＿＿＿＿＿＿＿＿＿＿＿＿＿＿＿＿

＿＿＿＿＿＿＿＿＿＿＿＿＿＿＿＿＿＿＿＿＿＿＿＿＿＿＿＿＿＿＿＿＿＿

2. About Expressions

Can you make a dialogue of taking a blood measure for wards?

Caregiver:_____

_____

_____

_____

_____

_____

_____

_____

3. Self-reflection

Can you share what you have thought in your learning process with us?

_____

_____

_____

_____

_____

_____

_____

_____

_____

_____

4. Quick Assessment

Read each statement in the table below and place a check mark in the column that best describes how well you can complete that task.

Subjects	Very hard	Hard	A Little Hard	No Problem	Great
I can read the passage by myself.					
I can understand the main idea of the text.					
I can finish tasks with my classmates.					
I can remember the new words and expressions.					
I enjoy myself in learning.					

Unit 2　Aging Population
老龄人口

Section A

Warm-up Activity【仁爱于心　健康与行】

Video 5–4

Let's Fill the Blanks

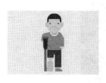 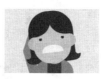 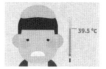

(1) She _____ something bad, so she is _____.

(2) It's going to _____ before he can _____.

(3) He needs to drink _____ of _____.

plenty,　food,　aches,　liquids,　enough

(4) She has a _____ in the back of her _____.

pain,　fever,　head,　plenty,　throat

(5) She doesn't _____ good because her throat _____.

pain,　feel,　sore,　hurts,　head

Key 5–3

Section B

Ⅰ Passage: Aging Population in China 【放眼世界　聚焦中国】

Graphics: Is China Ready for an Aging Population?

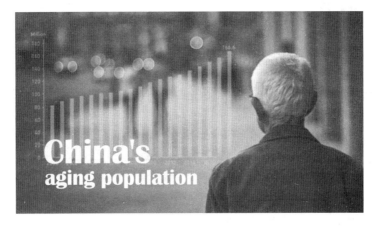

China, the most populous country in the world, is facing the rapid graying of its population.

At the end of 2018, 11.9 percent of its population (166.6 million people) were 65 or older, according to data from China's National Bureau of Statistics. Generally, a society is considered relatively (相对地) old when the proportion of the population aged 65 and over exceeds 8 to 10 percent.

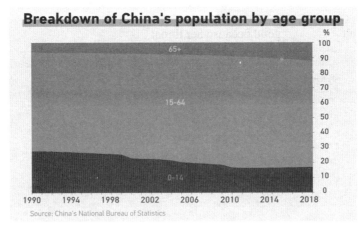

Breakdown of China's population by age group

Source: China's National Bureau of Statistics

The ratio of young to old will be dramatically (显著地) imbalanced by the rising ranks of the elderly. Seen from the graphic below, China's age dependency ratio (抚养比) for over 65 surpassed the world average's in 2009 and became three percentage points higher in 2018.

The age dependency ratio of older dependents is the proportion (比例) of people older than 64 to the working-age population, between 15 and 64.

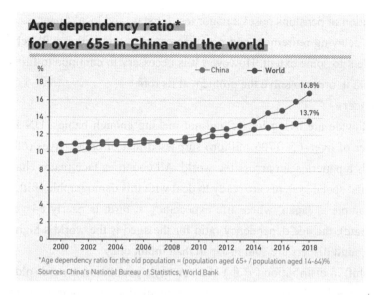

Age dependency ratio*
for over 65s in China and the world

*Age dependency ratio for the old population = (population aged 65+ / population aged 14-64)%
Sources: China's National Bureau of Statistics, World Bank

If we take a closer look at different regions in China, the whole country has entered (进入) an aging stage, but at distinct (清晰的) levels.

In southern Guangdong Province, for example, the age dependency ratio for the elderly is 10.3 percent, meaning 10 people in working age (14-64) support one senior citizen. Guangdong also has the largest GDP in China. However, in southwestern Chongqing Municipality, which had the highest age dependency ratio for the elderly in 2017, five young people need to support one elderly person.

Challenges and China's Response

China's aging crisis is well underway. Given the declining fertility (富裕) rate, China's aging process is irreversible and increases pressure in areas like pensions (养老金) and health systems.

China has taken measures to deal with the aging population, including building and improving medical and health systems for the elderly, promoting flexible (灵活的) retirement, encouraging family care combined with social care, and loosening birth policy.

Regions where the aging population is becoming a severe issue have already started to find different strategies to try and balance the situation, such as in Liaoning Province, where retirees are encouraged to start private businesses.

Reforming the birth control policy has so far done little to defuse China's aging issue.

China formally scrapped its one-child policy in 2016, and has since encouraged couples to have a second child—but the number of births has not surged as expected.

After a bump in 2016-consisting mainly of women who'd waited to have a second child-the birth rate then fell the following year. Many factors can influence a country's birth rates, including the number of women in fertility age, their educational level, and the overall social and economic development.

According to reports from the Chinese Ministry of Finance, China's pension expenditure has exceeded its collected premiums, and is largely relying on financial subsidies. Maintaining the smooth operation of pensions poses a major test for state and local finances.

Experts say delaying retirement and pensions entering the market will help to alleviate the current predicament to some extent. However, it is necessary to continue to further the reform of the pension system in order to solve the problem at its root.

Shared Concern

People worldwide are living longer and not making enough babies. UN figures show that the global number of over-65s (705 million) surpassed that of under-fives (680 million) at the end of 2018. It is a pattern seen across the world. All countries face major challenges to ensure that their health and social systems are ready to deal with this demographic shift.

A prime example is Japan, where life expectancy at birth is nearly 84 years (the world's highest national rate), the age dependency ratio for the aged is the world's highest, and the birth rate is low. More adult diapers are sold in Japan than infant ones.

While this shift in distribution (分布) of a country's population towards older ages started in high-income countries like Japan, it is now low-and middle-income countries that are experiencing the greatest changes. The World Health Organization expects that by the middle of the century many countries, including China, will have a similar proportion of older people to Japan.

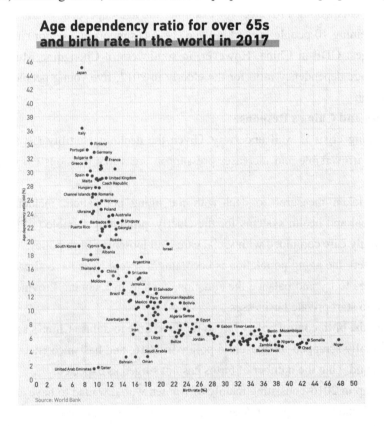

Healthy Aging

Older people are often assumed (假定) to be frail (瘦弱的) or dependent and a burden to society, which can lead to discrimination, affect the way policies are developed and the opportunities older people could have.

Population experts warn that policies promoting (促进) elderly health need to play a crucial part in mitigating the effects of aging populations, arguing that healthier individuals are more able to continue working for longer and with more energy, which could result in lower healthcare costs.

China still has a long way to go coping with (应对) its aging population. What's certain is that the clock for the "aging time-bomb" keeps ticking, calling for immediate action.

(*Source:* HAYOM News, 15 July 2019)

II Notes【说文解字 名词注释】

1. Vocabulary Table

Vocabulary 5–2

Words & Expressions	Part of Speech	Meaning in Text
relatively	*adv.*	相当程度上;相当地;相对地
dramatically	*adv.*	戏剧地;显著地
dependency ratio	*n.*	比例
proportion	*n.*	份额;比例
enter	*v.*	进入
distinct	*adj.*	明显的;清楚的
fertility	*n.*	富饶;富裕
pension	*n.*	养老金
flexible	*adj.*	灵活的;机动的
diaper	*n.*	尿布;尿片
distribution	*n.*	分布
assume	*v.*	假定;假设
frail	*adj.*	瘦弱的;弱的
promote	*v.*	促进;推动
cope with	*phr.*	积极应对;应对

2. Read Following Me

(1) How to read a passage?

Step 1   Find the key sentence of each paragraph.

Step 2   Divide the passage into 3 parts.

Step 3   Write down the main idea of each part.

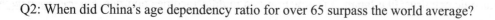
Key 5–4

Step 4   Answer the following questions.

Q1. What kind of society can be considered old according to the passage?

_____.

Q2: When did China's age dependency ratio for over 65 surpass the world average?

_____.

Q3: What challenges did China meet facing aging crisis?

_____.

Q4: What measures did China take?

_____.

Q5: What facts can affect a country's birth rate?

_____.

(2) How to read a sentence?

① China, the most populous country in the world, is facing the rapid graying of its population.

Step 1   China is facing the graying.

中国正面临银发族。

Step 2   China is facing the *rapid* graying *of its population*.

中国正面临快速人口老龄化。

Step 3   China, *the most populous country in the world*, is facing the rapid graying of its population.

中国,这个世界最大的人口大国,正面临快速人口老龄化。

② Seen from the graphic below, China's age dependency ratio for over 65 surpassed the world average's in 2009 and became three percentage points higher in 2018.

Step 1   China's *age dependency ratio* surpassed the average's and became higher.

中国的年龄抚养比超过了平均水平,并且越来越高。

Step 2   China's age dependency ratio *for over 65* surpassed *the world* average's in 2009 and became *three percentage points* higher *in 2018*.

2009年中国65以上的老年抚养比超过世界平均水平,并且比2018年高了3个百分点。

Step 3   *Seen from the graphic below*, China's age dependency ratio for over 65 surpassed the world average's in 2009 and became three percentage points higher in 2018.

从下图可以看出,2009年中国65岁以上的老年抚养比超过世界平均水平,并且比2018年提高了3个百分点。

③ While this shift in distribution of a country's population towards older ages started in high-income countries like Japan, it is now low-and middle-income countries that are experiencing the greatest changes.

Step 1   While this shift started in high-income countries, it is now low-and middle-income countries.

虽然这一转变始于高收入国家,但现在是中低收入国家。

Step 2   While this shift *in distribution of a country's population* started in high-income countries *like Japan*, it is now low-and middle-income countries.

虽然一国人口分布的这种转变始于日本等高收入国家,但目前正是中低收入国家。

Step 3   While this shift in distribution of a country's population *towards older ages* started in high-income countries like Japan, it is now low-and middle-income countries *that are experiencing the greatest changes*.

虽然一个国家的人口分布向老年人的转变始于像日本这样的高收入国家,但现在正是中低收入国家经历着最大的变化。

(3) How to read words and expressions?

Step 1　About the population.

The percent of population, the proportion of the population, dependency ratio, the fertility rate, the aging population, the number of births, distribution of population.

Step 2　About measures.

Reform the birth control policy, one-child policy, pension expenditure, pension system, health and social system, cope with aging population, promote elderly health.

🩺 Section C

Ⅰ Extensive Learning【深度学习　优游岁月】

Things to Do When You Retire

We sometimes find ourselves dreaming about our life after retirement since it marks a significant change and a new stage in our lives. While it is a scary (吓人的) thought for many; Some people take retirement as an opportunity to do things that they were unable to do while they were working.

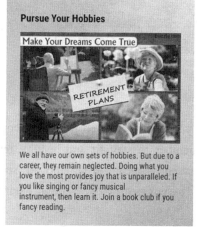

Pursue Your Hobbies

Make Your Dreams Come True

RETIREMENT PLANS

We all have our own sets of hobbies. But due to a career, they remain neglected. Doing what you love the most provides joy that is unparalleled. If you like singing or fancy musical instrument, then learn it. Join a book club if you fancy reading.

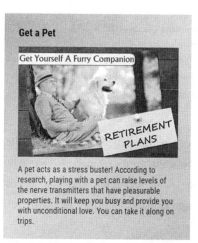

Get a Pet

Get Yourself A Furry Companion

RETIREMENT PLANS

A pet acts as a stress buster! According to research, playing with a pet can raise levels of the nerve transmitters that have pleasurable properties. It will keep you busy and provide you with unconditional love. You can take it along on trips.

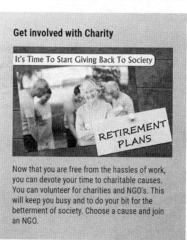

Get involved with Charity

It's Time To Start Giving Back To Society

RETIREMENT PLANS

Now that you are free from the hassles of work, you can devote your time to charitable causes. You can volunteer for charities and NGO's. This will keep you busy and to do your bit for the betterment of society. Choose a cause and join an NGO.

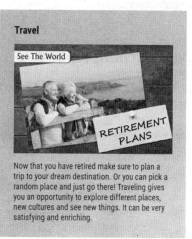

Travel

See The World

RETIREMENT PLANS

Now that you have retired make sure to plan a trip to your dream destination. Or you can pick a random place and just go there! Traveling gives you an opportunity to explore different places, new cultures and see new things. It can be very satisfying and enriching.

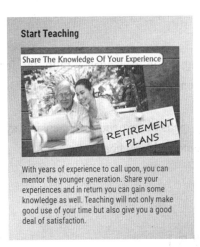

Start Teaching

Share The Knowledge Of Your Experience

RETIREMENT PLANS

With years of experience to call upon, you can mentor the younger generation. Share your experiences and in return you can gain some knowledge as well. Teaching will not only make good use of your time but also give you a good deal of satisfaction.

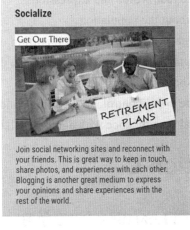

Socialize

Get Out There

RETIREMENT PLANS

Join social networking sites and reconnect with your friends. This is great way to keep in touch, share photos, and experiences with each other. Blogging is another great medium to express your opinions and share experiences with the rest of the world.

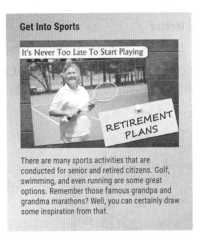

Get Into Sports

It's Never Too Late To Start Playing

RETIREMENT PLANS

There are many sports activities that are conducted for senior and retired citizens. Golf, swimming, and even running are some great options. Remember those famous grandpa and grandma marathons? Well, you can certainly draw some inspiration from that.

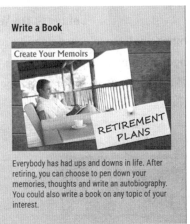

Write a Book

Create Your Memoirs

RETIREMENT PLANS

Everybody has had ups and downs in life. After retiring, you can choose to pen down your memories, thoughts and write an autobiography. You could also write a book on any topic of your interest.

Always keep a notepad and pen down the things you always wanted to do but couldn't because of time constraints (约束条件). Always remember to stay fit and healthy through regular exercise. And, just relax and take it easy. Retirement is meant to be enjoyed, so make sure that you make list of "things to do in retirement" as positive (积极的) and exciting as possible.

(*Source:* wellnesskeen.com)

Ⅱ Extensive Learning【拓展学习　岗位应用】

1. How to Test Your Blood Sugar（Video 5-5）

Video 5-5

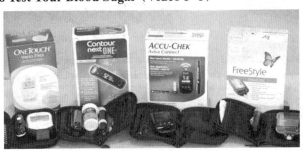

Preparation for Necessary Items 用物准备:

A blood sugar meter 血糖仪

A test strip (chech expiry date) 试纸

A lancing device 取血笔

A lancet 取血针

Cotton balls or tissues 棉签或消毒棉

A sharps container 便携式锐器盒

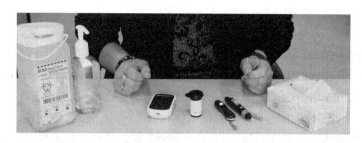

Steps 步骤:

Prepare to Test Your Blood Sugar Level:

(1) Wash hands. 洗手。

(2) Prepare the lancing device. 取出采血针。

(3) Remove the divice cap by twisting it off. 拧开采血针盖子。

(4) Insert a lancet into the holder. 把采血针装置插入针头固定处。

(5) Twist off the protective disk. 拧开采血针头的保护盖。

(6) Replace the divice cap. 把采血针盖子盖好。

(7) Adjust the depth setting (small er numbers = shallower puctures). 调试刺针深度 (数字小＝深度浅)。

(8) Insert a test strip into the meter. 将试纸插入血糖仪。

Lance Your Finger and Draw Blood for Testing:

(1) Choose a spot to lance your finger. 选择手指入针区域。

(2) Lance your fingership. 采血。

(3) Massage your finger in the direction of your fingertip. 挤压手指使血液至指尖处。

(4) Touch and hold the test strip opening to the drop. 用试纸测血糖。

Use Your Blood Sugar Meter:

(1) See the boold sugar's result on the meter's screen. 通过屏幕查看测试结果。

(2) Write the result on the bolld sugar's diary. 将测试结果记录在血糖记录本中。

(*Source:* Taipei City Foreign Caregivers Manual, 2014)

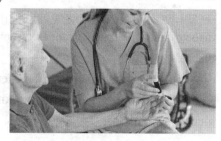

2. Blood Sugar Assessment

Nurse: Hello, Mr. Johnson. I just need to check your blood sugar, if that's OK? Please give me one of your fingers. 您好，约翰逊先生，我需要给您测血糖，可以吗？请伸出一根手指。

Patient: OK. 好的。

Nurse: OK, you will just feel tiny prick on the finger. 好。手指上会有一点点刺痛。

Patient: ALL right. 好，没有关系。

Nurse: Thanks. Your blood sugar level is 6 millimoles per litre (mmol / L). It is among the normal range. 谢谢。你的血糖值为6，在正常值范围内。

Patient: That's nice. 太好了。

Nurse: How have your BSLs / sugars been? 你以前的血糖如何？

Patient: Pretty stable. In fact, I never goes higher than nine millimoles per litre (mmol / L). 挺稳的，从来没有超过9.

Nurse: That's nice. Please keep it. 不错，需要保持住。

Doctor: How have Mr. Robert's BSLs / sugars been? 罗伯特先生的血糖如何？

Nurse: His BSL is 22 millimoles per litre (mmol / L). 他的血糖值是22.

Doctor: That's not good. He needs an insulin infusion and also need to go onto hourly BSLs too. 不太好。他需要扎胰岛素，并且需要1小时测一次血糖。

Nurse: OK, I see. 好。

Nurse: Mr. Robert has just had another hypoglycaemic episode. We have given him some glucose and a sandwich. His BSL is now four point nine. 罗伯特先生刚刚低血糖了。我们给他补充了糖和一块三明治。他现在血糖是4.9。

Doctor: OK, I'll chart it. We can recheck his BSL again in an hour. 好。我会关注，一个小时内我们再测一次。

Notes：

(1) Before we take blood sugar of someone, we should make a simple assessment. 当我们在给患者测量血压之前，我们通常需要做一些简单的评估。

(3) How have your BSLs / sugars been? 您之前的血糖如何？

(4) Do you have any history of hypoglycaemic episode? 您曾经有低血糖吗？

(5) What is your blood pressure usually like? 您一般血压是多少？

3. Blood Sugar Level Ranges

Understanding blood glucose (葡萄糖) level ranges can be a key part of diabetes (糖尿病) self-management. Here is "normal" blood sugar ranges and blood sugar ranges for adults and children with type 1 diabetes, type 2 diabetes and blood sugar ranges to determine people with diabetes.

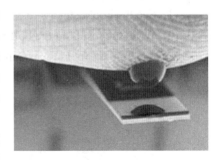

If a person with diabetes has a meter, test strips (测试条) and is testing, it's important to know what the blood glucose level means.

Recommended (推荐) blood glucose levels have a degree of interpretation (理解) for every individual (个人) and you should discuss this with your healthcare team. In addition, women may be set target blood sugar levels during pregnancy.

The following ranges are guidelines provided by the National Institute for Clinical Excellence (NICE) but each individual's target range should be agreed by their doctor or diabetic consultant (咨询).

Recommended Target Blood Glucose Level Ranges

The NICE recommended target blood glucose levels are stated below for adults with type 1 diabetes, type 2 diabetes and children with type 1 diabetes. In addition, the International Diabetes Federation's target ranges for people without diabetes is stated. The table provides general guidance. An individual target set by your healthcare team is the one you should aim for.

Target Levels by Type	Upon Waking	Before Meals (Pre Prandial)	At Least 90 Minutes After Meals (Post Prandial)
Non-diabetic*		4.0 to 5.9 mmol / L	under 7.8 mmol / L
Type 2 diabetes		4 to 7 mmol / L	under 8.5 mmol / L
Type 1 diabetes	5 to 7 mmol / L	4 to 7 mmol / L	5 to 9 mmol / L
Children w / type 1 diabetes	4 to 7 mmol / L	4 to 7 mmol / L	5 to 9 mmol / L

*The non-diabetic figures are provided for information but are not part of NICE guidelines.

Normal and Diabetic Blood Sugar Ranges

For the majority of healthy individuals, normal blood sugar levels are as follows:

Between 4.0 to 5.4 mmol / L (72 to 99 mg / dL) when fasting.

Up to 7.8 mmol / L (140 mg / dL) 2 hours after eating.

For people with diabetes, blood sugar level targets are as follows:

Before meals: 4 to 7 mmol / L for people with type 1 or type 2 diabetes.

After meals: under 9 mmol / L for people with type 1 diabetes and under 8.5mmol / L for people with type 2 diabetes.

Blood Sugar Levels in Diagnosing Diabetes

The following table lays out criteria for diagnoses (诊断) of diabetes and prediabetes.

Blood Sugar Levels in Diagnosing Diabetes			
Plasma GlucoseTest	Normal	Prediabetes	Diabetes
Random	Below 11.1 mmol / l Below 200 mg / dl	N / A	11.1 mmol / l or more 200 mg / dl or more
Fasting	Below 5.5 mmol / l Below 100 mg / dl	5.5 to 6.9 mmol / l 100 to 125 mg / dl	7.0 mmol / l or more 126 mg / dl or more
2 hour post-prandial	Below 7.8 mmol / l Below 140 mg / dl	7.8 to 11.0 mmol / l 140 to 199 mg / dl	11.1 mmol / l or more 200 mg / dl or more

Why are good blood sugar levels important?

It is important that you control your blood glucose levels as well as you can as too high sugar levels for long periods of time increases the risk of diabetes complications developing.

Diabetes complications are health problems which include:

kidney disease (肾病);

nerve damage (神经损伤);

retinal disease (视网膜疾病);

heart disease (心脏病).

This list of problems may look scary but the main point to note is that the risk of these problems can be minimized through good blood glucose level control. Small improvements can make a big difference if you stay dedicated (献身) and maintain those improvements over most days.

(*Source:* Diabetes.co.uk, 2019)

🩺 Section D

Projects in Practice【实践探索　行动项目】

1. Project 1

Make a dialogue: Practice blood sugar assessment with your classmates like caregivers and wards.

Caregiver: Hello, Mr. Johnson. I need to check your blood sugar, if that's OK? Please give me one of your fingers.

Ward: OK.

Caregiver: OK, you will feel tiny prick on the finger.

Ward: All right.

...

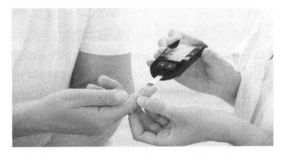

2. Project 2

Scene play: Take blood sugar for some of your classmates, teachers, family members or friends before diet in the morning and write them down.

Name	Age	Record	Low	Normal	High	Very High
Li Lingling	19	5.5 mmol / 1 100		✓		

3. Project 3

Understand the blood sugar levels.(Video 5−6)

Video 5−6

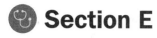 **Section E**

Self-assessment【进阶评估　自我超越】

1. About Words and Phrases

How many new words and phrases have been committed in your memory? Please write them down.

(1) Aging population: _____

_____

_____

(2) Senior citizen: _____

_____

_____

(3) Blood Sugar: _____

_____

_____

2. About Expressions

Can you make a dialogue of taking a blood sugar for wards?

Caregiver: _____

_____

_____

_____

_____

_____

3. Self-reflection

Can you share what you have thought in your learning process with us?

_____

_____

_____

_____

_____

_____

_____

_____

Chapter 5　Elderly Care

4. Quick Assessment

Read each statement in the table below and place a check mark in the column that best describes how well you can complete that task.

Subjects	Very Hard	Hard	A Little Hard	No Problem	Great
I can read the passage by myself.					
I can understand the main idea of the text.					
I can finish tasks with my classmates.					
I can remember the new words and expressions.					
I enjoy myself in learning.					

Unit 3　Activities for Senior Citizens

银发社区

⚕ Section A

Warm-up Activity【守护健康　乐享生活】

Video 5–7

1. Choose the Right Answer

Q1: Who can't work without crutches? _____

Q2: Who ate something bad? _____

Q3: Who has a soar throat? _____

Q4: Who has a pain in the back for the head? _____

Q5: Who has a fever? _____

2. Listen to the Sentence and Write Them Down

(1) _____.

(2) _____.

(3) _____.

(4) _____.

Key 5–5

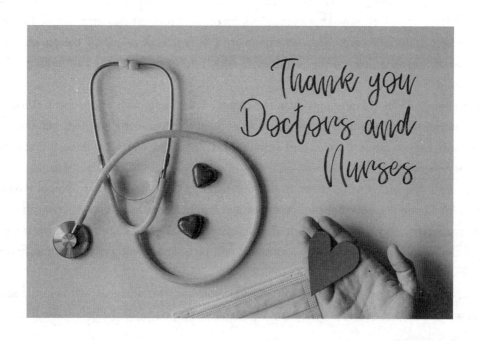

Section B

Ⅰ Passage: Activities for Senior Citizens【老有所乐　畅享生活】

Activities for Senior Citizens to Keep the Mind and Soul Healthy

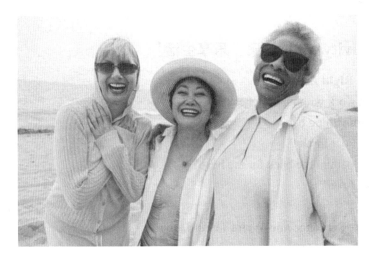

A lot of emphasis is put on keeping ourselves fit and occupied while we are in our salad-days (青少年时代). But, we should spare a thought about our old-age as well. It is the stage in which we need maximum attention and it is the stage in which we can very well become a couch potato (泡在电视机前的人). While working for as a customer service agent for a U.K.-based online-shopping company, I was impressed with the zeal (热情) and enthusiasm with which senior (较年长的人) citizens kept themselves involved. From art and craft items, to hot-air balloons, their attitude towards life was exemplary (典范). That is one of the reasons why I thought of writing an article on the activities in which our senior citizens can indulge (沉迷) themselves in.

Mix about 200 small safety pins in an ice-cream bucket along with dry oatmeal. Blindfold a person and time them for around 10 minutes and let them see how many pins they can find in the dry oatmeal. Let everyone have a turn (blindfolded), and the one who finds the maximum number of pins, wins a prize.

Pick up some inexpensive items from your local grocery store. Good choices would be toiletries, kitchen items, personal care products, and home decorations. These items can also be gift-wrapped as mystery prizes. You will also require some fake (假的) money, which is equally distributed along the participants. The auctioneer will pick up a single prize at a time, and start the bidding.

Everyone is supposed to get their own fishing pole and bait along. It will help the seniors relax as well as keep themselves occupied. There should be prizes for the maximum fish caught and the biggest catch.

Organize a yoga (瑜伽) class. This is extremely beneficial to senior citizens, and each person should do only those yoga exercises that they are comfortable with. However, this activity needs care and caution.

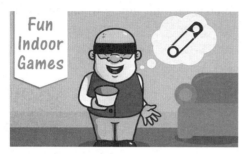 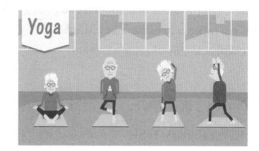

Some Other Activities for Seniors

Organize a one-mile walk. This is something which is within the capability of most senior citizens.

Mental exercises like solving puzzles and doing mathematical calculations without using a paper and pencil could be undertaken (实施). This might delay the onset of serious old age diseases like Alzheimer's, or delay the progress of the disease in people already afflicted (折磨) by this disease.

Monthly birthday parties can be a good way for senior citizens to catch-up with each other. Also, it will make the birthday a memorable experience.

Have a quiz regarding movies, songs, TV shows, actors, and other categories that the seniors are familiar with or are enthusiastic about.

Playing Favorites—We guess each person's favorite choices, for example, their favorite sport, favorite food, or favorite music genre. Keep prizes for those who guess it right and win.

Sculpting (雕刻) for seniors—You could use the soft clay products, which are made for children. There should be a prize for the quickest sculpture created and the best looking sculpture. This activity would also help in strengthening the seniors' dexterity and muscle control.

A holiday trip to a scenic spot could be organized. Nature is one of the most effective healers (缓解形势的事物) for the mind.

Hold a flower decoration (装饰) competition (比赛). Supply the flowers, vases, and scissors. You are allowed to take your handmade creation home.

Supply the seniors with cameras. Each one can take pictures of their favorite items, and display (展示) them to others as a slide show.

You could also place your favorite recipe among many recipes, and ask the seniors to guess it. Each senior can talk for a few minutes offering (主动提出) personal advice and tips on health-related issues.

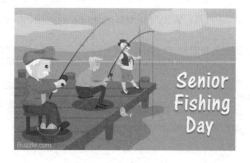

These were some activities for seniors. As we mentioned before, it is very important that senior citizens keep themselves occupied with some of the other activity, otherwise life can get a bit monotonous. Not only will these activities keep the senior citizens busy, these will also help them in being healthy and spontaneous (自然的). We hope that this article would be useful to everyone, especially our senior citizens.

(*Source:* wellnesskeen.com, 2008)

Ⅱ Notes【说文解字　名词注释】

1. Vocabulary Table

Vocabulary 5-3

Words & Expressions	Part of Speech	Meaning in Text
salad-day	*n.*	冒冒失失锋芒毕露的青少年时代
couch potato	*n.*	老泡在电视机前的人
zeal	*n.*	热情;激情
senior	*n.*	较……年长的人
exemplary	*adj.*	典范的
indulge	*v.*	沉湎;沉迷
fake	*adj.*	假的
yoga	*n.*	瑜伽
undertake	*v.*	负责
afflict	*v.*	折磨;使痛苦
sculpt	*v.*	雕刻;雕塑
healer	*n.*	缓解情势的事物
decoration	*n.*	装饰
competition	*n.*	比赛;竞赛
display	*v.*	陈列;展出;展示
offer	*v.*	主动提出
spontaneous	*adj.*	自然的;自发的

2. Read Following Me

(1) How to read a passage?

Step 1　Divide the passage into 3 parts.

Step 2　Write down the main idea of each part.

Step 3　Answer the following questions.

Key 5-6

Q1. Why did the author write the passage?

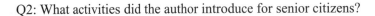

Q2: What activities did the author introduce for senior citizens?

Q3: What is the key to design activities for senior citizens?

Q4: Why it is important for senior citizens to take part in activities?

_____.

Q5: What's your view on keeping mind and soul healthy for senior citizens?

_____.

(2) Follow me: How to read a sentence?

① Let everyone have a turn (blindfolded), and the one who finds the maximum number of pins, wins a prize.

Step 1　Let everyone have a turn.

让每个人都有一个回合.

Step 2　Let everyone have a turn, _and the one wins a prize_.

让每个人都有一个回合,赢得一个奖。

Step 3　Let everyone have a turn (_blindfolded_), and the one _who finds the maximum number of pins_, wins a prize.

让每个人都有一个回合(蒙上眼睛),谁找到最大数量的针,赢得一个奖。

② It will help the seniors relax as well as keep themselves occupied.

Step 1　It will help the seniors.

这将有助于老年人。

Step 2　It will help the seniors _relax_.

这将有助于老年人放松。

Step 3　It will help the seniors relax _as well as keep themselves occupied_.

这将有助于老年人放松和保持自己的忙碌。

③ Mental exercises like solving puzzles and doing mathematical calculations without using a paper and pencil could be undertaken.

Step 1　Mental exercises could be undertaken.

可以进行心理练习。

Step 2　Mental exercises _like solving puzzles and doing mathematical calculations_ could be undertaken.

可以进行解谜和数学计算之类的心理练习。

Step 3　Mental exercises like solving puzzles and doing mathematical calculations without using a paper and pencil could be undertaken.

不需要纸和铅笔就可以进行解谜和数学计算之类的心理练习。

(3) Follow me: How to read words and expressions?

Step 1　About senior citizens.

Salad-day; couch potato; senior citizen; the attitude toward life.

Step 2　About activities.

Safety pin; kitchen item; keep oneself occupied; be beneficial to; care and caution; a one-mile walk; muscle control; flower decoration; handmade creation; health-related issue.

Section C

Ⅰ **Enhanced Learning**【深度学习 "玩"转大脑】

Games for Seniors to Boost Their Memory While Having Fun

Memory games not only help senior citizens improve their memory but also alleviate (缓和) loneliness, and, to an extent, reduce their health problems. Many brain - related health problems such as Alzheimer's (阿尔茨海默病), dementia (老年痴呆症) and anxiety could be controlled or reduced with memory games.

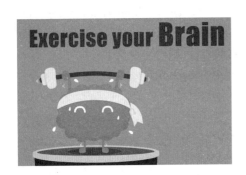

Forgetfulness, although a sad fact, is a part of old age. Statistics show that around 75% of seniors are concerned about their memory - related problems. Lapse (失效) of memory is not a disease, but an inevitable part of growing old. However, it can be reduced to a certain extent by engaging in brain exercises and memory games. One of the most interesting solutions to this problem is to constantly play memory - related games, which would help to keep the brain fit. Seniors, like kids, love to play games. Some of the popular games that many senior citizens play, even today, are card games, bingo, Scrabble and Uno.

An elderly, who has a memory problem, could improve his memory by challenging his

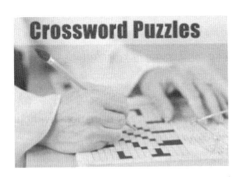

mind with puzzles, reading books, solving crossword, and playing other brain - exercising games. If you have grandchildren at home, take time out to play games with them. This would not only keep you mentally fit but also would be a good stress buster (破坏者). You may not believe but popular games like checkers, chess and monopoly help to improve the long-term as well as the short-term memory of seniors.

Crossword Puzzles

One of the best and most popular memory games for seniors is the crossword puzzle. You can either play it alone or ask one of your friends or spouse to join you. You can always use a dictionary for solving the puzzle. A crossword not only enhances (提高) your vocabulary skills but also keeps you mentally alert. There are many other

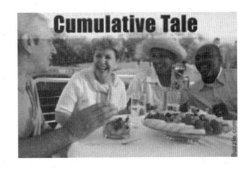

types of puzzles on the Internet which will also be helpful.

Cumulative Tale

One of the party games seniors could play is a cumulative (累积的) story-telling game. In this game, senior should sit in a circle. One of them should begin the game by saying, "On Monday, I had chicken sandwiches for dinner" The second person would repeat the line said by the earlier member and also add a

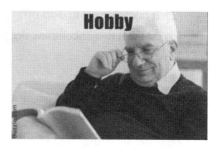

successive line. Continue the game till it comes back to the first person. He has to tell the original line, plus the successive lines added by other members.

Hobby

Take the popular game show 'Name That Tune' as a cue for creating an interesting memory game for seniors. You can play music or just the tune (曲调) on the music player or the karaoke (卡拉 OK) machine. Ask the group of seniors to identify the tune. The group can also sing the entire song together (after identification) to have more fun. Similarly, as an alternative, short clips of popular movies can be shown to people and asked to identify them.

It would be a wise idea to pursue (追求) a hobby that requires concentration. For instance, reading, a game of chess or solving a puzzle would mean racking your brain. This would enable you to retain your memory and enhance mental capabilities. Similarly, gardening, arts and crafts also provide the required exercise for brain.

Name the Things

You could ask a senior to take a look at one of his favorite rooms, for instance, his bedroom for a minute. Ask him to leave the room. Now, when the person comes out, ask him to describe the room; the color on the walls, the arrangement (安排) of the furniture, other noticeable things, etc. Similar game can be played by showing a picture card to a senior for a minute; and asking him to describe it. This is a fun game to improve one's memory.

There are reports to prove that the mnemonic (助记符) capabilities of an elderly person are most active in the early hours of the morning, decline throughout the day, and are least active as evening sets in. As you grow old, you should take up various activities along with your senior friends. These activities revitalize (使恢复) memory and can also be fun.

(*Source:* Wellnesskeen.com, 2008)

II Extensive Learning【拓展学习　岗位应用】

Video 5-8

1. How Aging Really Affects Your Sleep? (Video 5-8)

Here are 4 ways your sleep changes overtime, plus how to get the rest of you.

(1) Your clock shifts back.

Your body naturally moves toward earlier bed and wake times.

Tips:

Work out in the afternoon.

Exercise in the afternoon or early evening can help shift your body clock.

(2) It takes longer to drift off.

Experts call this "nocturnal sleep lantency (睡眠灯)," and it's common with age.

Tips:

Get better at bedtime.

Wind down with herbal tea, a warm bath and a good book. And shut down those screens.

(3) Napping gets easier.

Daytime snoozing comes faster with each passing year.

Tips:

Keep naps short.

Rest 20 minutes or less.

Too much daytime sleep can get in the way of your nighttime slumber (沉睡).

(4) There's less deep sleep.

70-year-olds get about half the deep sleep of younger adults.

Tips:

Watch what you drink and not just caffeine.

Alcohol may leave you drowsy, but can trigger midnight wakeups.

Sleeping less? It may be OK. Everyone's needs are different and change over time. Talk to your doctor about any concerns.

(*Source:* sleepfoundation.org, 2019)

2. The Connection Between Yoga and Better Sleep for Older People

Yoga isn't just beneficial for improving core strength, flexibility (灵活性), and stress levels; it can also help you sleep better—especially if you suffer from insomnia. When people who have insomnia perform yoga on a daily basis, they sleep for longer, fall asleep faster, and return to sleep more quickly if they wake up in the middle of the night. This is also true for older people who have insomnia (失眠) —those who are 60 and older experience better sleep quality, sleep for longer, and feel better during the day when they perform regular yoga.

This benefit can be seen in all sorts of situations where people have trouble sleeping. For example, pregnant women who start a mindful yoga practice in their second trimester (学期) sleep better and wake up less often throughout the night, and cancer patients sleep better if they do yoga (90 percent of cancer patients experience insomnia symptoms while receiving treatment).

If you want to work yoga into your bedtime routine, it's important to do the right kind. Some types of yoga can be energizing (like hot yoga and vigorous vinyasa flow), which won't help you relax as well as restorative styles of yoga like hatha and nidra. Here are three poses that are ideal for preparing your body for sleep.

(1) Legs Up the Wall: Lie on the ground on your back and put the back of your legs up a wall (keep your legs straight), so your body is in an L-shaped pose. Relax into the position, hold it for at least 30 seconds and focus on your breathing.

(2) Lying Butterfly: Lie on the ground on your back. Press the bottoms of your feet against each other and let your knees fall out to the sides. You can put a pillow under your knees if this feels too strenuous.

(3) Corpse Pose (挺尸式) : Lie on the ground on your back with legs straight, arms by sides, and palms facing up. Breathe slowly, focusing on your inhales and exhales.

(*Source*:sleepfoundation.org, 2019)

3. How to Make a Sleep Study

Your doctor will likely recommend a sleep study if the cause of your insomnia is unclear.

Medical History

To find out what's causing your insomnia, your doctor may ask whether you:

(1) have any new or ongoing health problems;

(2) have painful injuries or health conditions, such as arthritis (关节炎);

(3) take any medicines, either over-the-counter (非处方药) or prescription;

(4) have symptoms or a history of depression, anxiety, or psychosis;

(5) are coping with highly stressful life events, such as divorce or death.

Your doctor also may ask questions about your work and leisure habits. For example, he or she may ask about your work and exercise routines; your use of caffeine (咖啡因), tobacco, and alcohol; and your long-distance travel history. Your answers can give clues about what's causing your insomnia.

Your doctor also may ask whether you have any new or ongoing work or personal problems or other stresses in your life. Also, he or she may ask whether you have other family members who have sleep problems.

Sleep History

To get a better sense of your sleep problem, your doctor will ask you for details about your sleep habits. Before your visit, think about how to describe your problems, including:

(1) how often you have trouble sleeping and how long you've had the problem;

(2) when you go to bed and get up on workdays and days off;

(3) how long it takes you to fall asleep, how often you wake up at night, and how long it takes to fall back asleep;

(4) whether you snore loudly and often or wake up gasping or feeling out of breath;

(5) how refreshed you feel when you wake up, and how tired you feel during the day;

(6) how often you doze off (打瞌睡) or have trouble staying awake during routine tasks, especially driving.

To find out what's causing or worsening your insomnia, your doctor also may ask you:

(1) whether you worry about falling asleep, staying asleep, or getting enough sleep;

(2) what you eat or drink, and whether you take medicines before going to bed;

(3) what routine you follow before going to bed;

(4) what the noise level, lighting, and temperature are like where you sleep;

(5) what distractions, such as a TV or computer, are in your bedroom.

To help your doctor, consider keeping a sleep diary for 1 or 2 weeks. Write down when you go to sleep, wake up, and take naps. (For example, you might note: Went to bed at 10 a.m.; woke up at 3 a.m. and couldn't fall back asleep; napped after work for 2 hours.)

Also write down how much you sleep each night, as well as how sleepy you feel throughout the day.

You can find a sample (样本) sleep diary in the National Heart, Lung, and Blood Institute's "Your Guide to Healthy Sleep."

(*Source*: webmd.com, 2018)

Section D

Projects in Practice【实践探索　行动项目】

1. Project 1

Design an activity for senior citizens: Design a fun indoor game for senior citizens. Write down how to play and what to care and caution.

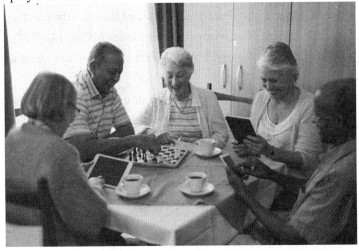

An Activity for Senior Citizens

_____

_____

_____

_____

_____

_____

_____

2. Project 2

Scene Play: Design a questionnaire for sleeping according to the passage "How to Make a Sleep Study".

Here is an example:

A Questionnaire About Food

(1) Which kind of food do you prefer?（   ）

A. Chinese food

B. Western food

(2) What your favorite food?（   ）

A. American chocolate cookies

B. Greek cheese pies

C. Indian curries

D. Chinese fried rice

E. Japanese sushi

F. Italian pizza

G. South African beef curry

3. Project 3

Senior activities at the community center.（Video 5-9）

Video 5-9

Section E

Self-assessment【进阶评估　自我超越】

1. About Words and Phrases

How many new words and phrases have been committed in your memory? Please write them down.

（1）Aging population: _____

_____

_____

（2）Senior citizen: _____

_____

_____

（3）Indoor activity: _____

_____

_____

2. About Expressions

Can you introduce one or two indoor games for senior citizen?

(1) _____

_____

_____

_____

(2) _____

_____

_____

_____

_____

3. Self-reflection

Can you share what you have thought in your learning process with us?

_____

_____

_____

_____

_____

_____

_____

_____

_____

_____

4. Quick Assessment

Read each statement in the table below and place a check mark in the column that best describes how well you can complete that task.

Subjects	Very Hard	Hard	A Little Hard	No Problem	Great
I can read the passage by myself.					
I can understand the main idea of the text.					
I can finish tasks with my classmates.					
I can remember the new words and expressions.					
I enjoy myself in learning.					

Unit 4   Attitudes Toward Elderly Care
长者照护

Section A

Warm-up Activity【增强体魄　行动起来】

Listen to the Sentences and Write Them Down.

(1) She _____ something bad, so she is _____.

(2) It's going to _____ before he can _____.

(3) He needs to drink _____ of _____.

(4) She has a _____ in the back of her _____.

(5) She doesn't _____ good because her throat _____.

Video 5–10

Key 5–7

Section B

Ⅰ Passage: Attitudes Toward Elderly Care【长者之家　民生关注】

Aging Society Brings Change in Attitudes toward Elderly Care

What will happen when you get old? That is a question more ordinary Chinese have found themselves contemplating (考虑).

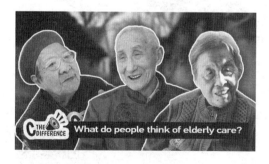

91 - year - old Li has made herself a new home in an elderly - care community inside a quadrangle courtyard, tucked away in an old - fashioned Beijing alleyway. She told CGTN that her only son, who lives in coastal Shenzhen in the south, doesn't know she's here. "He is away. I don't tell him anything," Li said, while sitting outside in the sun with other residents (居民) of the care home.

On this early spring day, the courtyard had a rare serenity (宁静) that contrasted (与……对比) with the city life outside. And the residents were in good spirits.

Xing, 88, has lived here for four years. He commended (赞扬) the care home's staff for keeping the place clean and tidy, and said he is in good health. "Students at the nearby primary school would come and visit us. It's so great to see them," Xing grinned (咧开嘴笑).

Zhang agrees that she is well taken care of. "He (my son) worried that I would fall or bump into something," said the 83-year-old, who walks with a crutch (腋杖). "The staff here cook us hot meals that are served on the table. It's good."

The Golden Fall Garden elderly-care home belongs to the local community and is now managed by a private firm specializing (专门研究) in elderly care services. The quadrangle courtyard has been modified (调整) to be more friendly to seniors.

The so-called "silver economy" (银发经济) of providing products and services for the elderly is booming (迅速发展) in China. The industry is expected to double its size from 2018 to reach 8 trillion yuan in 2020, or about 7 percent of China's GDP. Experts widely agree that elderly care is a "rising sun industry."

The Chinese have a tradition of raising children who would in turn care for parents in old age. Until the past decade, nursing homes and commercial elderly care were considered novel (新颖的) concepts for many Chinese families. But that is going to change, and soon.

After four decades of the one-child policy, China's single-child generations, who make up the majority of its working population, are finding it increasingly difficult to care for elderly family members and their own offspring (子女). More Chinese seniors are checking themselves into nursing homes.

"I don't want to live with my children. I asked them and said whether they agree or not, I must live here," said Wu. Her two sons visit her every week, as long as they have time off, she told CGTN, showing pictures of her family at the care home.

In recent years, upmarket nursing homes incorporating healthcare and hospitality facilities (设备) have sprouted (涌现出) across the country, offering an appealing (吸引) vision of what retirement life could be.

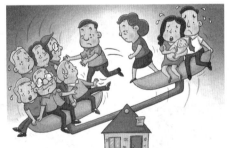

"The nursing homes that I saw are all modern. I was extremely surprised to see inside them," a woman in her early 20s who didn't give her name told CGTN. "The elderly are enjoying their lives. My husband and I would be very happy to live there," she said

(*Source:* CGTN News, April 5, 2019)

Ⅱ Notes【说文解字　名词注释】

1. Vocabulary Table

Vocabulary 5-4

Words & Expressions	Part of Speech	Meaning in Text
contemplate	*v.*	考虑;思量
resident	*n.*	居民
serenity	*n.*	宁静;平静
contrast	*v.*	对比;对照
commend	*v.*	(尤指公开地)赞扬;称赞;表扬

Words & Expressions	Part of Speech	Meaning in Text
grin	*v.*	露齿而笑;咧着嘴笑
crutch	*n.*	(腿或脚受伤病人用的)腋杖
specialize	*v.*	专门研究(或从事)
modify	*v.*	调整;使更适合
silver economy	*n.*	银发经济
boom	*v.*	迅速发展;激增
novel	*adj.*	新颖的;与众不同的
offspring	*n.*	子女;后代
facility	*n.*	设施;设备
sprout	*v.*	(使)涌现出
appeal	*v.*	吸引

2. Read Following Me

（1）How to read a passage?

Step 1　Find the key sentence of each paragraph.

Step 2　Divide the passage into 3 parts.

Step 3　Write down the main idea of each part.

Step 4　Answer the following questions.

Key 5-8

Q1. What question did more ordinary Chinese consider according to the passage?

_____.

Q2: What did those seniors living in local elderly-care home think about their life ? Did they satisfied with it? Why?

_____.

Q3: Why is "silver economy" booming according to the passage?

_____.

Q4: Why did more Chinese seniors check themselves into nursing homes?

_____.

Q5: What did Wu's attitude toward living in care home?

_____.

Q6: What did the modern nursing home like?

_____.

(2) Follow me: How to read a sentence?

① Zhang agrees that she is well taken care of.

Step 1　Zhang agrees.

张同意。

Step 2　Zhang agrees <u>that she is taken care of</u>.

张同意她<u>被照顾</u>。

Step 3　Zhang agrees that she is *well* taken care of.

张同意她受到<u>很好的</u>照顾。

② The staff here cook us hot meals that are served *on the table*.

Step 1   The staff cook us meals.

工作人员给我们做饭。

Step 2   The staff cook us meals *that are served*.

工作人员<u>为</u>我们<u>做了</u>饭菜。

Step 3   The staff *here* cook us *hot* meals that are served *on the table*.

<u>这里的</u>工作人员给我们做<u>餐桌上热腾腾的</u>饭菜。

③ The nursing homes that I saw are all modern.

Step 1   The nursing homes are modern.

养老院很现代化。

Step 2   The nursing homes *that ...* are modern.

<u>……的</u>养老院都很现代化。

Step 3 The nursing homes *that* I saw are *all* modern.

<u>我看到的</u>养老院<u>都</u>很现代化。

(3) Follow me: How to read words and expressions?

Step 1   About the name of elderly care home.

The elderly-care community; the care home; silver economy; rising sun industry; the nursing home.

Step 2   About the life in elderly care home.

Keep the place clean and tidy, in good health/spirit, serve sb on the table, be friendly to seniors ; provide products and services for the elderly.

Step 3   About the single-child generation.

Care for parents in old age; the one-child policy; working population; have time off.

🩺 Section C

Ⅰ Enhanced Learning【深度学习　寻找记忆】

Brief Introduction of Alzheimer's Disease

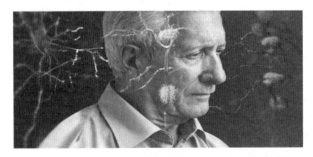

In 1901, a 51-year-old female August was admitted to the Frankfurt Hospital in Germany. According to her family members, she was suffering from the gradual decline of memory and understanding ability, and she couldn't talk as smoothly as before. Simultaneously (同时), she was stated to be illusive of listening inability of direct-making and identifying goods, and occasionally to be paranoid.

After Dr. Alzheimer taking a comprehensive examination and some supporting treatment, the symptoms (症状) of August hadn't seen any improvement but rather to be worse.

5 years later, Dr. Alzheimer reported this case in the annual conference of Psychiatry held in Germany. She firstly named this disease as a strange cortical related disease, manifesting (显化) as severely decline of restoring message and decline of time and location navigational ability.

In the following years, Dr. Alzheimer biopsied the brain tissue of the patient, and she found the wide atrophy of brain and its volume (容量) reduced. Through microscope, she found the cortex (皮层), as well as the sub-cortical gray matter (皮质下灰质), showed a widespread breakdown of neural cells, the proliferation of gliocyte (胶质细胞增殖), entanglement (纠缠) of neural fibers (神经纤维) and plaques of silver-staining (银染斑块).

In 1910, the 8th edition of textbook Psychiatry name the symptoms above after Dr. Alzheimer as Alzheimer's Disease, for short as AD.

Manifestation "A-B-C"

A refers to Activity, which indicates the reduced ability to complete activities of daily living.

B refers to Behavior, which indicates behavioral and psychological symptoms of dementia, such as depression, anxiety, illusion, delusion, and insomnia etc. in psychological aspect and pacing, attacking, wandering, fidget and screaming etc. in behavioral aspect.

C refers to Cognition, which indicates the decline of cognition (认知). The initial typical symptom is memory disorder, manifesting as recent memory impairment while the long-term one is still normal. The patient may repeatedly forget the latest events and communication, familiar names but can easily tell stories when he/she was young.

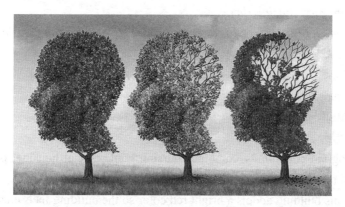

Sometimes, these symptoms may be ignored by being considered as complications (难题) of aging but may gradually develop to daily activities and can't speak clearly and smoothly, even can't calculate the navigate.

Unfortunately, AD patients will suffer two deaths, one is mentally and the other is physical, which bring a lot burden to both patients and family to endure.

(*Source: YiXueSheng*, 3 Jan. 2018)

II **Extensive Learning【拓展学习　岗位应用】**

The Design of an Elderly Community

What would be your first impression when someone mentions that they are sending their loved ones to an Elderly Community? In this article, we will review 4 senior housing examples from different parts of the world and see what inspirations we can learn from them.

Elderly Communities in Europe

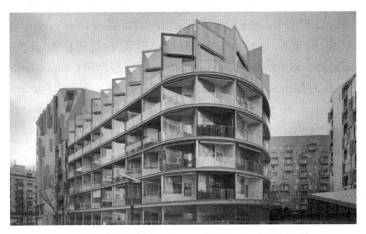

A Nursing House, Clichy-Batignolles, Paris, France

Design Firm: Atelier du Pont.

Location: Paris, France.

Community's Category: Nursing House.

Marketing Advantage: This project was a response to the elevated need for housing in the area.

Number of Beds: 129 beds.

Surfaces: 6,117 m².

Color: Red, Orange, White, Brown.

Special Material: Wood and lots of glass.

Completed in 2015.

This multi-program community combines nursing home, social housing, private housing, religious center, and retail stores.

The facade of this building adopts a bright red color so the building feels energetic, which is important for elderly people. In addition, the rooms have large open windows in multiple directions, which increases both the brightness in their rooms and the interaction between the indoor space and the neighborhood environment. The entire building feels urbanish (类城市化) from the top to the bottom.

Besides, each room in the community has its own outdoor balcony, and the architects used glass materials to bring the environment and the natural light closer to the residents. The natural environment reduces loneliness and social isolation among elder residents.

Some people like to live in an urban, while others would prefer living closer to nature. For the second type of people, this nursing home, locating at the foothills of the "Wilder Kaiser" Mountain Range, might suit their tastes.

Elderly Communities in Austria

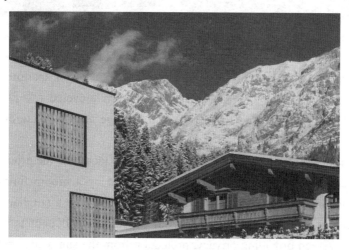

Wilder Kaiser Retirement and Nursing Home, Australia

Design Firm: Dürschinger Architekten, SRAP Sedlak Rissland.

Lead Architects: René Rissland, Uli Wiese.

Location: Austria.

Community's Category: Nursing House.

Marketing Advantage: Great location, directly adjacent to a former residential and care home that no longer corresponds to the required standards.

Number of Beds: 54 apartments (around 100 beds).

Surfaces: 5,120 m².

Color: Yellow, Green, White, Brown, Black.

Special Material: Wood and lots of glass on the roof.

Completed in 2017.

Located close to the Mountain Range and the Village Centre of Scheffau, this Retirement Nursing Home, "Wilder Kaiser", was opened at Dec 2017. It is made up of 2 buildings and 3 public areas—a public garden, a separate dementia garden, and a playground for children.

The public areas are located on the ground floor level. Close to the Main Entrance are the Café-Lounge, Event Hall and the Chapel. In the rear of the ground floor, there are the administrative offices, service rooms, and a production kitchen.

The interior and exterior spaces offer enough possibilities for private contemplation (沉思). The central and green atrium brings daylight inside the building. Furthermore, it enables visual communication across floors, between the dining areas, and communal areas of the different care units.

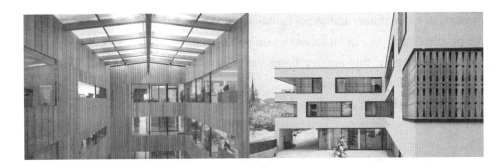

These Units are spread over the two upper levels with a total of 54 apartments. Smaller community spaces are situated throughout a care group with cantilevered (悬臂式), roofed terraces (梯田) and balconies, orientated to the Mountain Range and the picturesque Village Centre of Scheffau.

Wooden framework made of untreated larch emphasizes the facade of the ground floor and the recessed balconies. The rest of the outer surface is covered by a broom finished plaster. Wooden inlays of profiled larch boards accentuate the windows. They are a familiar reference to local handcrafted traditions. But the traditional system of cutouts and palings is translated contextually and used as screen providing privacy, protection from the sun while painting subtle shadows on the facade.

Elderly Communities in China

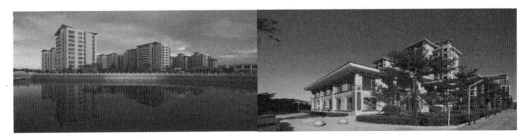

Yanda International Health City, Tianjin, China

Design Firm: Tianjin Yanda International Health City Investment Management Co., Ltd.
Location: Tianjin, China.
Community's Category: Home Health, Assisted Living, Nursing Homes, and Memory Care.
Marketing Advantage: It matches the large population (105,000,000) around Beijing.
Number of Beds: 9,500 beds (about 100 times larger the projects above).
Surfaces: 650,000 m² (about 100 times larger than the projects above).
Color: Yellow, Brown, Black.
Special Material: Marble and wood inside.
Completed in 2010.

To satisfy the huge population, there are several giant senior communities located in Beijing and its nearby areas, and "Yanda" is the one that stands out. The Yanda International Health Centre lies several kilometers east of Chaobai River, which borders Beijing and Hebei.

Yanda Health Center takes up about 150 acres. There are 1,500 beds in its first phase of the construction, with 90 percent of the residents from Beijing, and new 8,000-bed addition in the second phase projected to opening 2020. 6,000 beds of it have already been filled up.

Yanda has the golden age health care center, Hebei Yanda hospital (the first class hospital in China), elderly university, old-age service center, elderly rehabilitation rooms, community health service centers, a commercial center, a bilingual kindergarten, and a dormitory building. For the end-of-life (EOF) services, it has a Catholicism church, a Christian church, an Islam mosque, and a Buddhism temple. Thousands of older adults live here to enjoy their retirement lives.

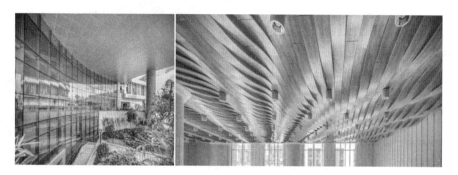

Senior Activity Center, Guangxi, China

Architect: Atelier Alter.
Location: Guangxi, China.
Community's Category: Senior Center.
Surfaces: 1,632 m².
Color: Orange, Yellow, White.
Material: Bamboo.
Completed in 2014.

The architecture design of the "Senior Activity Center" in Guangxi was intended for seniors who spent most of their youth in the Cultural Revolution period of China. Its bamboo-like wooden-aluminum exterior matches the classical ancient design of the local culture. The project tries to evoke that sense of belonging for our parents' generation.

The balcony would make a big difference for senior housing, however, with the amount of residents served in one Chinese community, balancing between a spacious private space and a gorgeous public area has always been difficult.

(*Source:* RuiRan RAN, 24 May. 2019)

Section D

Projects in Practice【实践探索 行动项目】

1. Project 1

Design an elderly community: Design an elderly community and picture them down.

Designer: _____

Location: _____

Community's category: _____

Marketing Advantage: _____

Number of Beds: _____

Surfaces: _____

Style: _____

Color: _____

Special Material: _____

Interior Area: _____

Public space: _____

2. Project 2

Fill the table: Read brief introduction of Alzheimer's Disease in section C and fill the following tables.

"A-B-C"	Menifestation	Symptom
A		
B		
C		

3. Project 3

A home for elderly healing.（Video5-11）

Video 5-11

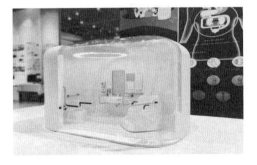
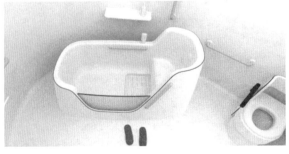

Section E

Self-assessment【进阶评估　自我超越】

1. About New Words and Phrases

How many new words and phrases have been committed in your memory? Please write them down.

(1) Elderly care house: _____

_____

_____

(2) Alzheimer's Disease: _____

_____

_____

2. About Expressions

Can you make a design of future elderly community?

沐浴区

如厕区

洗漱区

3. Self-reflection

Can you share what you have thought in your learning process with us?

_____

_____

_____

_____

_____

_____

_____

_____

_____

4. Quick Assessment

Read each statement in the table below and place a check mark in the column that best describes how well you can complete that task.

Subjects	Very Hard	Hard	A Little Hard	No Problem	Great
I can read the passage by myself.					
I can understand the main idea of the text.					
I can finish tasks with my classmates.					
I can remember the new words and expressions.					
I enjoy myself in learning.					

Chapter 6

Medical Professionalism and Globalization

国际医护

Unit 1　Health Care en Route: A Global Vision
"医"在旅途

Section A

Warm-up Activity【健康旅游　时尚潮流】

Share your opinion with your group members based upon the video "Seven Top Trends in Wellness Tourism 2019" (Video 6–1), and conclude your ideas with NO MORE than 20 words in English.

Video 6–1

Here is an example:

People are travelling overseas for health care services because of better or cheaper medical treatment abroad. (16 words)

Section B

Ⅰ Figures, Data and Facts【事实记录　数据呈现】

Young People Most Likely to Go Abroad Without Insurance

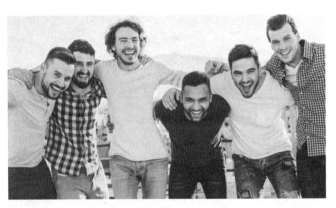

About 25% of British holidaymakers are thought to not buy travel insurance before going abroad.

About 40% of young people go abroad without travel insurance (保险), risking medical fees of thousands of pounds if they are taken ill, a survey suggests. The Association of British Travel Agents surveyed 2,043 Britons (英国人) and found those aged 18 to 24 were the most likely to go abroad without insurance. It comes after the family of a South Yorkshire traveller in Thailand had to raise £32,000 for his medical care. Overall a quarter of UK travellers are thought to go abroad without insurance.

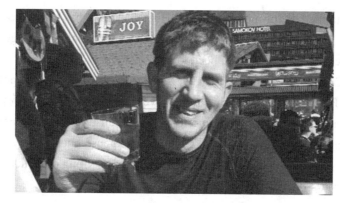

Craig Lindley was left paralysed in Thailand without travel insurance; his friends raised £32,000 towards his medical bills.

In 2015, 35-year-old Craig Lindley, from Barnsley, fell ill while celebrating a friend's wedding on a Thai (泰国的) island. He was diagnosed (诊断) with Guillain-Barré syndrome (综合征)-which affects the peripheral (周边的) nervous system—and was left paralysed (使瘫痪). He was charged £20,000 for a five-day course of treatment in Bangkok (曼谷). His ambulance (救护车) and speedboat from the island to Koh Samui Hospital also cost £17,000. After an online appeal (筹款) his family and friends raised £32,000 towards his medical bills. The Association of British Travel Agents' (Abta) Mark Tanzer said: "Rather than having to resort to (诉诸) the kindness of strangers, holidaymakers should make sure that they have the right insurance in place."

Overall, the number of British travellers surveyed without insurance has risen to 25% in the 12 months to May, up from 22% the previous year. Mr Tanzer added: "Every year, we see cases of people falling into difficulty due to travelling without insurance. Often their families have to raise thousands of pounds for their treatment or repatriation (回国) and that's why it is so worrying to see an increase in younger people travelling without insurance."

In 2016, Michael Doyle, 29, was admitted to a private hospital in Bulgaria (保加利亚) after being diagnosed with blood poisoning. He required dialysis (透析) treatment which he received in the hospital, but he passed away before his parents were able to raise about £20,000 required

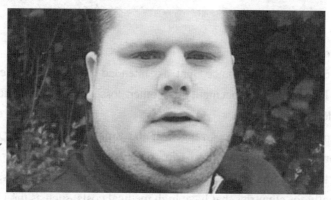

Michael Doyle was taken ill while in Bulgaria, his travel insurance would not cover a medical flight back to the U.K.

to bring him back to the UK for more treatment. His father John has advised people to get travel insurance. He said: "Go and enjoy yourself, Bulgaria is an excellent place to go, it's not different from anywhere else in the world but you need to have insurance."

Foreign and Commonwealth Office (FCO, 英国外交和联邦事务部) spokeswoman Susan Crown said: "The FCO cannot pay medical bills if you are hospitalised (送院治疗) abroad, nor can we fly you home. Take out an appropriate (合适的) insurance policy and make sure you know what it covers you for. It may feel like an added expense but it's very worthwhile if you compare it to what you could end up paying if something goes wrong on holiday."

(*Source:* BBC News UK, 20 May 2017)

II Notes【说文解字 名词注释】

Vocabulary 6–1

1. Vocabulary Table

Words & Expressions	Part of Speech	Meaning in Text
insurance	*n.*	保险;保费
Briton	*n.*	英国人
Thai	*adj.*	泰国的
diagnose	*vt.*	诊断(疾病)
syndrome	*n.*	综合病征;综合症状;症候群
peripheral	*adj.*	周围的;周边的;附带的
paralyse	*vt.*	(英式)使瘫痪;麻痹
Bangkok	*n.*	曼谷
ambulance	*n.*	救护车
appeal	*n.*	(慈善)筹款;呼吁;恳求
resort to	*phr.*	诉诸
repatriation	*n.*	遣返;回国
Bulgaria	*n.*	保加利亚
dialysis	*n.*	(医)透析
Commonwealth	*n.*	英联邦
hospitalise	*vt.*	(英式)将……送入医院治疗
appropriate	*adj.*	合适的;恰当的

2. Useful Knowledge

(1) Travel insurance is insurance that is intended to cover medical expenses, trip cancellation, lost luggage, flight accident and other losses incurred while traveling, either internationally or domestically.

Travel insurance can usually be arranged at the time of the booking of a trip to cover exactly the duration of that trip, or a "multi-trip" policy can cover an unlimited number of trips within a set time frame. Some policies offer lower and higher medical-expense options; the higher ones are chiefly for countries that have high medical costs, such as the United States.

Some credit card issuers offer automatic travel insurance if travel arrangements are paid for using their credit cards, but these policies are generic and particular care must be taken to take into account personal requirements. There are many travel insurance policies available in the market place, but care must be taken of what events are covered by each policy, and what exclusions, exceptions and limits apply, besides other issues.

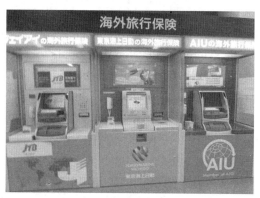

Travel insurance vending machines in Japan.

(2) South Yorkshire is a metropolitan county in England.

It is the southernmost county in the Yorkshire and the Humber region and had a population of 1.34 million in 2011. It has an area of 1,552 square kilometres (599 sq mi) and consists of four metropolitan boroughs, Barnsley, Doncaster, Rotherham and Sheffield. South Yorkshire was created on 1 April 1974. Its largest settlement is Sheffield.

(3) Tourism is a major economic contributor to the Kingdom of Thailand.

Estimates of tourism revenue directly contributing to the Thai GDP of 12 trillion baht range from one trillion baht (2013) 2.53 trillion baht (2016), the equivalent of 9% to 17.7% of GDP. When including indirect travel and tourism receipts, the 2014 total is estimated to be the equivalent of 19.3% (2.3 trillion baht) of Thailand's GDP. The actual contribution of tourism to GDP is lower than these percentages because GDP is measured in value added not revenue. The valued added of the Thailand's tourism industry is not known (value added is revenue less purchases of inputs). According to the secretary-general of the Office of the National Economic and Social Development Council speaking in 2019, the government projects that the tourism sector will account for 30% of Thailand's GDP by 2030, up from 20% in 2019.

As of 2019, with 64 accredited hospitals, Thailand is currently among the top 10 medical tourism destinations in the world. In 2017, Thailand registered 3.3 million visits by foreigners seeking specialised medical treatment. In 2018, this number grew to 3.5 million. As of 2019 Thai medical centres are serving increasing numbers of Chinese medical tourists in tandem with increasing overall Chinese tourism. All numbers reported by the government must be viewed with some skepticism according to the authors of a 2010 study. The Thai government reported that in 2006, 1.2 million medical tourists were treated in Thailand. But the 2010 study of five private hospitals that serve more than 60% of foreign medical tourists concluded that there were 167,000 medical tourists in Thailand in 2010, far below the government estimate. Most came for minor elective (cosmetic) surgery.

(4) Guillain-Barré syndrome (GBS) is a rapid-onset muscle weakness caused by the immune system damaging the peripheral nervous system.（吉兰-巴雷综合征又称格林巴利综合征，是以周围神经和神经根的脱髓鞘病变及小血管炎性细胞浸润为病理特点的自身免疫性周围神经病。）(Video 6-2)

Video 6-2

The initial symptoms are typically changes in sensation or pain along with muscle weakness, beginning in the feet and hands. This often spreads to the arms and upper body, with both sides being involved. The symptoms develop over hours to a few weeks. During the acute phase, the disorder can be life-threatening, with about 15% developing weakness of the breathing muscles requiring mechanical ventilation. Some are affected by changes in the function of the autonomic nervous system, which can lead to dangerous abnormalities in heart rate and blood pressure. The cause is unknown.

(5) In medicine, dialysis is the process of removing excess water, solutes, and toxins from the blood in people whose kidneys can no longer perform these functions naturally. This is referred to as renal replacement therapy. Dialysis is used in patients with rapidly developing loss of kidney function, called acute kidney injury (previously called acute renal failure), or slowly worsening kidney function, called Stage 5 chronic kidney disease, (previously called chronic kidney failure and end-stage renal disease and end-stage kidney disease). Dialysis is used as a temporary measure in either acute kidney injury or in those awaiting kidney transplant and as a permanent measure in those for whom a transplant is not indicated or not possible. In Australia, the United Kingdom, and the United States, dialysis is paid for by the government for those who are eligible. The first successful dialysis was performed in 1943.

(6) Bulgaria is a member of the European Union, NATO, and the Council of Europe; it is a founding state of the Organization for Security and Co-operation in Europe (OSCE) and has taken a seat on the UN Security Council three times. Its market economy is part of the European Single Market and mostly relies on services, followed by industry-especially machine building and mining-and agriculture.

(7) The Foreign and Commonwealth Office (FCO), commonly called the Foreign Office (which was the formal name of its predecessor until 1968), or British Foreign Office, is a department of the Government of the United Kingdom. It is responsible for protecting and promoting British interests worldwide and was created in 1968 by merging the Foreign Office and the Commonwealth Office. The head of the FCO is the Secretary of State for Foreign and Commonwealth Affairs, commonly abbreviated to "Foreign Secretary".

Section C

I Enhanced Learning【深度学习　关注沟通】

Nicole Pajer is sharing with the readers her experience dealing with a medical emergency while travelling abroad. Read through the passage and understand the importance of communication in health care.

Twenty-three hours. That's how long it was going to take us to get back home from Egypt. The journey would involve four airplanes: Aswan to Cairo, Cairo to Paris, Paris to New York, New York to Los Angeles. Plus one 45-minute Uber ride to get to our front door. This was the calculation I was running in my head when trying to decide what to do about the blood clot I was convinced was in my leg.

I'll admit: Too much reading on random medical websites got me to this panicked line of thinking. I lay in the bed at our hotel in Aswan, clutching my phone close while reading through symptoms of blood clots.

Have you been inactive for hours upon end? Yes. Three planes to get to Egypt, frequent naps in the hotel to overcome jet lag, a ferry boat Nile River cruise, a three-hour car ride each way to visit the breathtaking temple of Abu Simbel on the border of Sudan...

On our first day in Egypt, I hiked up the exterior of the Great Pyramid. I made it up the intensely steep staircase inside to the center—I had trained for months so I could do it. When I returned to the hotel where we were staying in Cairo that evening, I fell into bed with an unwavering satisfaction. "I did it!" I exclaimed to my half-asleep husband.

Our next adventure was a Nile River cruise. But as it went on, I noticed that my left calf was getting progressively more sore. The pain worsened every day, and it wasn't long before I found myself wincing with every step up the long staircase between our boat's dining room and our bedroom on board. After arriving at our last stop of Aswan, my calf was tender to the touch, swollen, and the pain had radiated up my whole leg.

When my husband was a child, his father died suddenly from a blood clot, so that's always been in the back of my head. You've probably heard or read the recommendation to get up and move around on long flights when you can, and I'm typically pretty good at doing this. But I was trapped in the middle seat with a passenger who rarely got up on my longest of three flights on the way to the Middle East and had thus been too lazy to follow my typical routine. So when the pain arose, I was completely convinced that I had developed a blood clot, and it had only worsened as we went along.

At this point, we were in Aswan, which is a city about 540 miles south of Cairo on the Nile River and seemed to me a bit less bustling than the capital city of Cairo. I was completely unfamiliar with the area and had no idea where the nearest hospital was, but I knew that I needed to be seen before I could physically get home. I went down to the lobby of the hotel and asked if they had a doctor on site. They did, but he wouldn't be available until the following evening. The hotel staff recommended that I visit a local German hospital, and said I could get there in a cab. The hospital wasn't presently open but would reopen in the morning. So we set our alarms for 5 a.m. the next day, got up, and hailed a cab.

Once we spotted the hospital's red cross sign, I approached the check-in window. But I wasn't prepared with much Arabic, so it was tricky for me to convey what was wrong with me to the staff at the counter. He asked me to pay a small admittance fee before handing me a piece of paper with Arabic writing on it and motioning for me to sit in the waiting area.

When it was my turn to be seen, a nurse directed me to a station, where I hopped onto a scale. The next steps were typical of a visit to the doctor: I got my temperature taken, gave a urine sample, etc. Slowly, I began to get better at acting things out. Although I didn't speak the language, it was amazing to witness our ability to communicate in other ways. I tried my best to say shukran (thank you) as often as possible. Though the staff giggled at my terrible accent, everyone seemed to appreciate the effort. I wanted to be as respectful—as "good" a tourist—as I possibly could be.

A nurse brought me in to see an English-speaking German doctor who did an ultrasound and determined that I did not in fact have a blood clot. The verdict was that I had pulled a muscle, possibly due to the way I had been favoring my left leg for the duration of the trip by leading with my left foot. (I now babied the right side of my body after sustaining my hip injury a year back.) He gave me the all-clear and wrote me a script for an anti-inflammatory medication, should I need it.

Thankfully, I wasn't dealing with any severe health issues. But the situation was admittedly stressful. I was in pain and in a foreign country. I had no idea how things would work in terms of insurance and payments; I just knew I needed my leg looked at. I didn't speak the local language. In hindsight, I should have been better prepared.

(*Source:* Nicole Pajer, 15 April 2019)

II Extensive Learning【拓展学习　媒体动态】

"Foreigners abusing system" claim contradicted by research that also shows more people go overseas for treatment than arrive.

Medical tourism is a lucrative source of income for the NHS, according to a major new study that contradicts many of the assumptions behind the government's announcement that it will clamp down on foreigners abusing the health service.

Eighteen hospitals—those deemed most likely to be making money from overseas patients—earned £42 m in 2010, according to researchers from the London School of Hygiene and Tropical Medicine and York University. Medical tourists spent an estimated £219 m on hotels, restaurants, shopping and transport in the U.K.

Read more from
The Guardian, 2013

When Melissa Moore travelled from the US to Costa Rica for knee replacement surgery she decided to keep it a secret.

"I didn't tell my friends and family because I didn't want them to say 'are you crazy?'," says the 53-year-old.

"Of course I also had my own misgivings about travelling to Central America and having major surgery."

Melissa, from the town of Brandon in Mississippi, is one of a growing number of people around the world who are going abroad for cheaper or quicker medical treatment.

While many Americans do so because they don't have health insurance—official figures show that more than 28 million do not—others like Melissa go overseas because their basic cover means that they have to pay a sizeable chunk of any treatment bill.

Read more from
BBC Business, 2019

Read more 6-2

A number of ministries responded to a series of public concerns over the past week, including public healthcare insurance, tourism and government procurements.

Another 36 expensive medicines have been added to the list of public healthcare insurance coverage, according to a notice recently released by the Ministry of Human Resources and Social Security.

With subsidies from healthcare insurance, the average prices of those medicines has dropped by 44 percent, compared to those in 2016, the notice said.

Some medicines will be sold at only 30 percent of last year's price. Imported medicines will sell less than in surrounding economies, significantly reducing medical bills for patients.

On the list are 31 Western medicines and five Chinese, taken to alleviate diseases such as lung cancers and kidney ailments.

Read more from
China Daily, 2017

Read more 6-3

While most travellers aim to stay out of the hospital while on vacation, a growing number of people are crossing international borders for the purpose of attaining medical services.

Widespread air travel, mounting healthcare costs in developed countries, long waiting lists and an ageing world population have all contributed to a global explosion of medical tourism in the past decade—and Asia is leagues ahead in terms of world market share.

More than 89% of medical tourists travelled to Thailand, India or Singapore in 2010, with Bangkok and Singapore leading the pack. But the cost of hotel rooms and treatment are both far more expensive in Singapore than in the Thai capital, making Bangkok the most popular place for medical tourism in the world. Even after the devastating floods of 2011, 19 million tourists visited Thailand in 2011, a 20% jump from 2010, with an estimated 500,000 travelling specifically for medical treatment, whereas of the 10.2 million tourists that visit Singapore each year, only 200,000 go to receive medical care.

Read more from
BBC Travel, 2012

Read more 6-4

Video Resources for Extensive Learning
(1) What is medical tourism? (Video 6-3)
(2) Access to medical services in Japan. (Video 6-4)

Video 6-3   Video 6-4

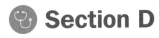 **Section D**

Projects in Practice【实践探索　行动项目】

1. Project 1

News Report: Read through the following passage and discuss within your group how to make hospital communication as clear as possible.

Dr. Pinckney suggests bringing an interpreter who speaks the local language to accompany you to the ER if you can. For instance, if you have a friend that you're visiting, Airbnb host, or perhaps a friend of a friend who speaks your language as well as the local language, they are good people to ask for help. Or, if you're staying at a hotel, you can ask the staff if they have someone available or inform the hospital front desk that you need assistance with language translation. You can also contact the International Medical Interpreters Association for assistance in locating one.

If these are not possibilities, be prepared to use a translator tool, Caitlin Donovan, director of outreach and public affairs for the National Patient Advocate Foundation, tells us. "You definitely don't want any miscommunication during a medical emergency," Donovan says. "If you're not fluent and don't have a human translator handy, use an app to ensure that you and your medical team understand each other." Google Translator is a good option, she says.

2. Project 2

Viewpoint: Over the years technology has been growing fast, some young people argue that international travelers no longer need to learn a foreign language, while others still believe that, in a globalized world, gaining a good command of a language other than one's mother tongue will help improve the experience during the stay abroad. What is your opinion?

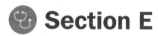 Section E

Self-assessment【进阶评估　自我超越】

1. Cooperative Learning Assessment

Please check your contribution to the group after the project is done.

	Superior (5)	Above Average (4)	Average (3)	Below Average (2)	Weak (1)
Understood what was required for the project					
Participated in the group discussion					
Helped the group to function well as a team					
Contributed useful ideas					
How much work was done					
Quality of completed work					
What could you improve upon next time?					
Your group members' comments					
Your group leader's comments					

2. Assessment of Individual Study

Instructions:

(1) Read each statement in the table below and place a check mark in the column that best describes how well you can complete that task.

(2) Review your responses for each task. If you have checked five or more in the "Somewhat" and / or "No" columns, you may need to consider making greater efforts after class.

I can	Yes	Somewhat	No
Understand the main idea of the text			
Identify the major points, important facts and details, and vocabulary in the text			
Make inferences about what is implied in the text			
Recognize the organization and purpose of the text			
Remember the new words and expressions			
Speak on the topic effectively			
Employ search strategy to gain information to address the project			
Refer to appropriate resources to deal with the project			

3. Personal Development

Instruction:

Completing this section will help you make informed practicing decisions. Please identify your strengths and the areas that you need to develop or strengthen and record them below.

STRENGTHS:
I am confident that I can...
(1)
(2)
(3)
AREAS FOR IMPROVEMENT:
I would like to improve my ability to...
(1)
(2)
(3)

Unit 2　Study Abroad as an International Student

海外学习

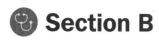 **Section A**

Warm-up Activity【家书寄语　留学感言】

An international student in the College of Nursing is writing an email to her parents after the first couple of days in the program. Watch the video "Advice for International Students in the College of Nursing"（Video 6-5）and discuss with your group members what difficulties she may encounter in the study, and what possible solutions she will find to address the challenges. Conclude your ideas with NO MORE than 20 words in English.

Here is an example:

Financial pressure seems a problem for some international students, but they may apply for the scholarships available on campus. (19 words)

Video 6-5

Section B

Ⅰ　Figures, Data and Facts【事实记录　数据呈现】

Philippines Seeks to Attract More Chinese Students

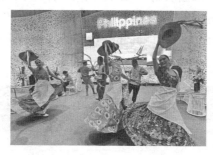

Performers danced at the Philippines' National Pavilion at the CIIE in Shanghai.

The Philippines' pavilion (菲律宾展馆) is one of the most eye-catching at the National Exhibition and Convention Center in Shanghai, the venue for the first China International Import Expo. (博览会) Designed to resemble an oyster (牡蛎) shell opening to reveal a luminescent pearl (明珠) —believed to be the first product Philippine traders exchanged with their Chinese counterparts—the whitewashed pavilion pays homage to bilateral (双边的) relations between the two nations that stretch back more than 400 years.

The Philippines also stands out because it is one of the few Southeast Asian nations at the expo that is not just offering tangible (有形的) products such as agricultural or electronic goods—it also wants to sell higher education. It's little surprise that the country is targeting the education sector. After all, China is the world's largest source of international students. According to the Ministry of Education, 608,400 Chinese students went overseas to study last year, marking the first time the figure had crossed the 600,000 mark, a rise of almost 12 percent from 2016.

But the odds (概率) look to be against Philippine universities, as Europe and the United States are still the most popular destinations for Chinese students, and higher education institutes in the Philippines are hardly renowned on the global stage. Only two—the University of the Philippines and De La Salle University—have made it into the 2019 World University Rankings compiled (编制) by Times Higher Education. Regardless, industry players from the Philippines are optimistic (乐观) of getting a slice of the pie. Their main selling points? Affordability and high-quality English courses.

"We are definitely cheaper than places like the US and the UK. In fact, we probably offer the cheapest English - language education in the world," said Leopoldo Valdes, senior internationalization officer at Holy Angel University in Angeles City, Central Luzon.

"Nearly everyone in the country speaks English. And we have what people call a 'neutral (中性) accent', which makes it easier for people to pick up and practice the language."

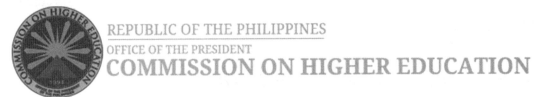

REPUBLIC OF THE PHILIPPINES
OFFICE OF THE PRESIDENT
COMMISSION ON HIGHER EDUCATION

Joy Christine Bacwaden, chief education program specialist at the Philippine Commission on Higher Education, said students are spoiled (宠坏的) for choice, as the country is home to some 2,000 higher education institutions. In addition to English courses, universities in the Philippines are also known for high - quality degrees in nursing and engineering, as well as hospitality (酒店业) and tourism, she added.

Higher Education Institutions in the Philippines in 2016 / 2017		
TYPE OF INSTITUTION	NUMBER	PERCENT OF TOTAL
Public	233	12%
State Universities and Colleges	112	-
Local Colleges and Universities	107	-
Other Government School	14	-
Private	1,710	88%
Total	1,943	100%

Source: Commission on Higher Education (CHED)
*Numbers do not include satellite campuses or extension centers.

 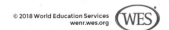

Jeremy Godofredo Morales, director of international relations at St. Paul University in Tuguegarao, said about 200 Chinese students have graduated from the school since 2005, and many are now working as nurses in hospitals in the United Kingdom, the US and Australia.

"We have always had Chinese students at our university. In fact, the Chinese connection even extends to our history. One of the co-founders of our university was a Chinese nun," he said.

(*Source: China Daily*, 09 Nov. 2018)

Ⅱ Notes【说文解字　名词注释】

Vocabulary 6-2

1. Vocabulary Table

Words & Expressions	Part of Speech	Meaning in Text
Philippines	*n.*	菲律宾
pavilion	*n.*	展馆;亭子
Expo	*n.*	展览会;博览会
oyster	*n.*	牡蛎;蚝
luminescent	*n.*	发光的;荧光的
pearl	*n.*	珍珠
bilateral	*adj.*	双边的
tangible	*adj.*	有形的;切实的;可触摸的
the odds look to be against	*phr.*	If you say that the odds(概率) are against something or someone, you mean that they are unlikely to succeed.
compile	*vt.*	编制;汇编
optimistic	*adj.*	乐观的
neutral	*adj.*	中立的;中性的
spoil	*vt.*	破坏;糟蹋;溺爱,宠坏
hospitality	*n.*	酒店服务;好客

2. Useful Knowledge

(1) Philippines has a simple literacy rate of 95.6%, with 95.1% for males and 96.1% for females. The Philippines had a functional literacy rate of 86.45%, with 84.2% for males and 88.7% for females in 2008.Spending on education accounted for 16.11% in the national budget proposed for 2015. Filipino and English are the official languages of the country. Filipino is a standardized version of Tagalog, spoken mainly in Metro Manila and other urban regions. Both Filipino and English are used in government, education, print, broadcast media, and business.

(2) The National Exhibition and Convention Center (Shanghai) (NECC), 国家会展中心 (上海), is an exhibition and convention centre in Shanghai, China. The NECC is currently the largest exhibition complex, making it one of the landmark buildings in Shanghai. The building was co-built by Ministry of Commerce of China and Shanghai Municipal Government. The center consists of four exhibition halls, the NECC Plaza, office buildings and a hotel. The facade

of the NECC building draws inspiration from a "four-leaf clover" with the plaza as the core and the exhibition halls as its leaves. Located in the Qingpu District in western Shanghai, the NECC enjoys multiple means of transportation provided by the Hongqiao transportation hub, including buses, metro, high-speed railway and airport. Metro Line 2's East Xujing station is the closest metro station to the center.

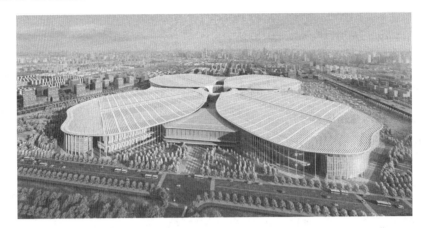

(3) According to the MOE (Ministry of Education, 教育部), the momentum in the number of Chinese students studying abroad and returning from overseas studies continued in 2017. Returning students are increasingly equipped with the skills required to support industrial development and government strategies for growth. 608,400 Chinese students left the country to pursue advanced studies overseas in 2017, tipping the number over the 600,000 mark for the first time, in an 11.74% increase on 2016 and cementing China's position as the world's largest source country for international students. The number of learners returning to China after completing their course reached 480,900, up 11.19% on the previous year, of which 227,400 with a master's degree or higher, up 14.90%.

Statistics show China has become the largest source of international students thanks to its growing pool of potential candidates. In total, 5,194,900 Chinese students have studied abroad over the last 40 years, and 1,454,100 students are currently enrolled in overseas higher education institutions. In 2017, while developed countries and regions, such as the U.S. and Western Europe, remained the most popular destinations, Belt and Road (B&R) countries have begun to harvest the growing wave of Chinese students seeking to learn abroad. In total, 66,100 students, including 3,679 on government sponsorships, studied in 37 B&R countries, highlighting this above-average growth of 15.7% since 2016.

(4) College and university rankings are rankings of institutions in higher education which have been ranked on the basis of various combinations of various factors. None of the rankings give a comprehensive overview of the strengths of the institutions ranked because all select a range of easily quantifiable characteristics to base their results on. Rankings have most often been conducted by magazines, newspapers, websites, governments, or academics. In addition to ranking entire institutions, organizations perform rankings of specific programs, departments, and schools. Various rankings consider combinations of measures of funding and endowment,

research excellence and/or influence, specialization expertise, admissions, student options, award numbers, internationalization, graduate employment, industrial linkage, historical reputation and other criteria.

The three longest established and most influential global rankings are those produced by ShanghaiRanking Consultancy (the Academic Ranking of World Universities; ARWU), Times Higher Education (THE), and Quacquarelli Symonds (QS). All of these, along with other global rankings, primarily measure the research performance of universities rather than their teaching. They have been criticised for being "largely based on what can be measured rather than what is necessarily relevant and important to the university", and the validity of the data available globally has been questioned.

(5) The history of nursing in the Philippines stems from the caregiving provided by women, priests, and herb doctors during precolonial Philippines. During the American period in the Philippines, Filipino women were given the chance to become educated as nurses, guided by their American nurse and missionary mentors, until nursing became a full-pledged profession in the Philippines, a professional career not only for modern-day women in the country but also for men in the Philippines (as male nurses). The advance of nursing in the Philippines as a career was pioneered by a culture of care which was intrinsic in the Filipino people. This was also the case even before Spanish colonization in communities. The way the health system was delivered also evolved.

The Philippines is the leader in exporting nurses to meet the demands of the United States and other developed nations. It has been argued, however, that the Philippines' persistent production of nurses for the global market is a state strategy to develop an export industry for economic development. Things such as immigration services and nursing licensing authorities encourage the production of nurses for export.

Of all registered health practitioners, nurses are among the largest group, even though there are very few nursing positions or jobs available to them. Only 15%—25% of jobs in the Philippines are provided for the nursing population. The remainder of the work force go on to seek out other professional career opportunities outside the country. Per year, the national government has approximately 18,000 nursing positions with an eventual turnover of 1,000 careers. The increase of Filipino nurses overseas has attracted the curiosity of other countries to better understand nursing in the Philippines and what makes Filipino nurses accommodating.

The first two years of general education is grounded on liberal arts that strengthen the values and character of the person as a caregiver. The language of instruction in all local institutions is English. This prepares the student for licensure both locally and internationally. This also gives the nurses access to ever - growing literature in the health sciences. The community skills, competence and confidence in the use of English certainly contribute to healthcare in any setting. The curriculum also strengthens the students' capabilities to participate in research in nursing and other health sciences, provides flexibility in the openness to the use of new teaching approaches, and encourages active involvement in extension work that reaches out to the other sectors. All registered nurses in the Philippines are required to have a bachelor's degree in nursing.

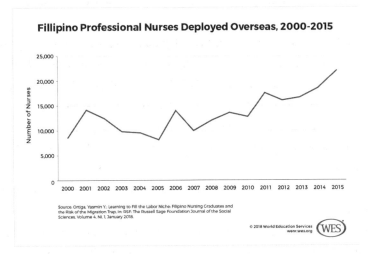

(6) Philippine English is any variety of English native to the Philippines, including those used by the media and the vast majority of educated Filipinos. English is taught in schools as one of the two official languages of the country, the other being Filipino (Tagalog). Due to the highly multilingual nature of the Philippines, code-switching such as Taglish (Tagalog-infused English) and Bislish (English infused with any of the Visayan languages) is prevalent across domains from casual settings to formal situations.

Today a certain Philippine English, as formally called based on the World Englishes framework of renowned linguist Braj Kachru, is a recognized variety of English with its distinct lexical, phonological, and grammatical features (with considerable variations across socioeconomic groups and level of education being predictors of English proficiency in the Philippines). As English language became highly embedded in Philippine society, it was only a matter of time before the language was indigenized to the point that it became differentiated from English varieties found in the United States, United Kingdom, or elsewhere.

Terminology related to education in the Philippines follow American usage, but there are also terms that are more or less unique to the Philippines: e.g. A minor subject is any elective or extra-curricular subject; A practicumer refers to a student who participates in a course of study that involves the supervised practical application of previously studied theory or an intern (which is frequently preferred). The word is coined from practicum, which means internship.

(7) A neutral accent is an accent that is not discernable as originating in any specific region. At present, there IS no neutral accent on a global level. That is, English accents are still divided into British, American, Australian, etc. However, within some of these accents, there are sub-accents that are considered "neutral". In British English, there is no neutral accent. Instead, there is a "standard" accent: Received Pronunciation, otherwise known as the Queen's English or BBC English. In American English, there IS a neutral accent called General American. Wikipedia states that "General American is perceived by most Americans to be 'accent-less', meaning a person who speaks in such a manner does not appear to be from anywhere."

While General American is not restricted to any one region in the United States, it is most commonly spoken in the Midland region. As such, the terms Midland accent and General American are often used synonymously. The Midland region covers parts of Illinois, Indiana, Iowa, Kansas, Missouri, Nebraska, and Ohio. When Americans attend an accent reduction class in an effort to eradicate their regional accents, they are taught the General American accent. This accent is commonly used by newscasters and actors, and according to Wikipedia, it is often considered "preferable to other regional accents." Furthermore, General American is often used when teaching English as a second language in schools worldwide (especially in Asia). It is the most commonly used English accent in the world today, and some linguists have argued that General American will eventually become the global neutral English accent.

Section C

I Enhanced Learning【深度学习　申请步骤】

Before Study Abroad: Applications, Fees & Visas

Here is an example if you are planning to be an international student in the Philippines.

Not only is the Philippines a beautiful country, it also has one of the best higher education systems in Asia, ranked 46th in the first edition of the QS Higher Education System Strength Rankings. Offering the opportunity to study in English at an affordable cost, the Philippines attracts over five thousand international students a year from across the globe, with most coming from other countries in East Asia. If you're fluent in English, you should be able to get by fairly well—English is one of the country's official languages and is widely spoken by residents, although less commonly outside of large cities.

Applying to Universities in the Philippines

There are two intakes for entry into universities in the Philippines, one in June and one in November. You should apply directly to your chosen university, providing an academic transcript relevant to your level of study. Depending on the university and program, you may also need to provide letters of recommendation and / or sit admission exams.

As the language of instruction at most universities in the Philippines is English, you'll need to prove your proficiency with a test such as IELTS or TOEFL if you're not a native speaker.

Applying for a Philippines Visa

All international students will need a student visa, which you'll need to apply for from the Philippine embassy or consulate in your home country after you've gained admission at a Filipino university. You'll need to provide the right documents (which should be stated on your embassy's website) and then attend an interview at the embassy or consulate. Your Philippines visa will be valid for a year and is renewable each semester. The documents you'll typically need include:

Your passport, which should be valid for at least six months after you intend to leave the Philippines;

Your completed visa application form;

A medical health certificate (DFA Form 11) with life-size chest x-ray and laboratory reports;

Three photographs of yourself;

A police clearing certificate;

Your notice of acceptance to study at a university in the Philippines;

Proof that you have enough money to support yourself during your stay, or a scholarship;

Your paid visa fee.

Fees and Funding

International students looking to study in the Philippines will be pleased to read that living costs are very low—you'll only need around US$4,200–US$6,000 per year. Tuition fees are also on the low side. Universities set their own fees and they will vary between programs, but you'll pay an average of US$1,000 per year at public universities and US$1,200 to US$2,500 at private institutions.

Note that your student visa does not allow you to find part-time work in the Philippines while you study, so you can't supplement your expenses as you go.

Health and Safety

You should secure health insurance before you study in the Philippines. You may be able to acquire this from the Philippine Health Insurance Corporation, which provides affordable health insurance for all citizens. However, you should also check the options available in your home country. It's also a good idea to visit your health professional before your visit to check if you need any vaccinations before you set off to the Philippines.

The Philippines' location on the Pacific 'Ring of Fire' makes it prone to earthquakes and typhoons, the latter of which can be expected during the rainy season from June to November. There are also numerous volcanoes in the Philippines. It's wise to read up on what to do in case of any natural disasters. As of April 2016, the island of Mindanao and the Sulu Archipelago are considered dangerous due to terrorist activity so visitors are not advised to visit these locations.

Ⅱ Extensive Learning【拓展学习　媒体动态】

According to the MOE, the momentum in the number of Chinese students studying abroad and returning from overseas studies continued last year.

Returning students are increasingly equipped with the skills required to support industrial development and government strategies for growth. 608,400 Chinese students left the country to pursue advanced studies overseas in 2017, tipping the number over the 600,000 mark for the first time, in an 11.74% increase on 2016 and cementing China's position as the world's largest source country for international students. The number of learners returning to China after completing their course reached 480,900, up 11.19% on the previous year, of which 227,400 with a master's degree or higher, up 14.90%.

Statistics show China has become the largest source of international students thanks to its growing pool of potential candidates. In total, 5,194,900 Chinese students have studied abroad over the last 40 years, and 1,454,100 students are currently enrolled in overseas higher education institutions. In 2017, while developed countries and regions, such as the US and Western Europe, remained the most popular destinations, Belt and Road (B&R) countries have begun to harvest the growing wave of Chinese students seeking to learn abroad. In total, 66,100 students, including 3,679 on government sponsorships, studied in 37 B&R countries, high-lighting this above-average growth of 15.7% since 2016.

Read more from
MOE, 2018

Read more 6-5

The Times Higher Education World University Rankings 2020 includes almost 1,400 universities across 92 countries, standing as the largest and most diverse university rankings ever to date.

The table is based on 13 carefully calibrated performance indicators that measure an institution's performance across teaching, research, knowledge transfer and international outlook.

The only university ranking to be independently audited by professional services firm PricewaterhouseCoopers, and trusted worldwide by students, teachers, governments and industry experts, this year's league table provides great insight into the shifting balance of power in global higher education.

For the fourth year in a row, the University of Oxford leads the rankings in first place, while the University of Cambridge falls to third. The California Institute of Technology rises three places to second, while Stanford, Yale, Harvard and Imperial College London all appear in the top ten.

Mainland China now provides both of Asia's top two universities, with Tsinghua and Peking universities finishing at 23rd and 24th place respectively. The country's universities have continued to expand their influence and presence on the world stage.

Read more from
Times Higher Education (THE), 2019

Read more 6-6

Candid self-appraisals lend weight to doubts about English capabilities of learners coming to Australia.

A new analysis has reinforced concerns about the English language skills of international students in Australian universities.

Tertiary education analyst Andrew Norton crunched data from Australia's 2016 national census to evaluate persistent claims about students' poor English skills. He tallied people's appraisals of their own English, restricting his analysis to answers from non-citizens who had arrived in Australia between 2014 and 2016 and were studying full-time at university.

Nine per cent of these respondents indicated that they did not speak English well. When the analysis was restricted to people from mainland China, that figure rose to 16 per cent.

Read more from

Times Higher Education (THE), 2019

Read more 6-7

The Philippines welcomes China's Belt and Road Initiative (一带一路), an ambitious effort to link Asia, Europe and Africa through the construction of massive infrastructure such as railways and ports, government officials and analysts have said.

Philippine Trade Undersecretary Ceferino Rodolfo said on Tuesday that the Belt and Road Initiative would help in advancing the socioeconomic programs of the administration of Philippine President Rodrigo Duterte.

"We welcome all international initiatives that would be consistent with (Duterte's) socio-economic agenda," Rodolfo told a news conference after the 28th Philippines-Chinese Joint Commission on Economic and Trade Cooperation.

The "belt" roughly with the historic Silk Road crossing Eurasia, while the "road" refers to the "maritime silk road"—the sea routes along which Southeast Asia, South Asia, Arabia and Africa traded with ancient China. Over the next 10 years, China aspires to achieve 2.5 trillion U.S. dollars in annual trade with the nations involved in the two areas.

Read more from

Xinhuanet, 2017

Read more 6-8

Video Resources for Extensive Learning
(1) International student experiences in nursing.（Video 6-6）
(2) Why not men in nursing?（Video 6-7）

Video 6-6   Video 6-7

Section D

Projects in Practice【实践探索　行动项目】

1. Project 1

Programme Prospectus: Read through the introduction to U.K. nursing courses, and discuss within your group if U.K. is the ideal destination for your further study.

International students wishing to register and work in the U.K. nursing profession are required to complete the Overseas Nursing Programme (ONP) as part of their studies. The ONP enables international students to become registered nurses in the U.K., where they are then registered to work in either the NHS or the private sector.

The ONP may be integrated as part of BSc (Hons) and MSc courses in International Nursing Studies and students can therefore gain an undergraduate/postgraduate degree in International Nursing Studies, obtaining registration with the Nursing and Midwifery Council (NMC) to work in the U.K. Each of these courses are full-time for one year, during which time students are given the option to undertake the ONP, which involves 400 hours of supervised practice placement. During study, international students studying at universities in the U.K. are permitted to work 20 hours per week during term time and full-time during holidays.

Most nursing degrees last for four years and students will cover a wide variety of the different aspects of Nursing during this time. Compulsory courses in life sciences will take place; while placements in various community and medical centres will enable students to gain firsthand experience of their profession. Lectures, tutorials, practical sessions and group work will cover each aspect of Nursing during study.

Careers in Nursing

Nursing graduates can focus on four separate areas during study—adult, child, learning disability and mental health—which will shape your future career. No two days for a fully qualified nurse are ever the same, and choosing what to focus on at the beginning of your career does not mean you are held in that particular environment permanently.

What do Nursing Graduates earn?

Average starting professional salary: £21,909

Average starting non-professional salary: £16,380

(*Source*: *The Times* and *Sunday Times Good University Guide*, 2019.)

Nursing U.K. Entry Requirements

Nursing is a very competitive area of study and it is important to not only show academic excellence when applying, but also have the right personality to take on such a demanding role. Students must have good numeracy and literacy skills, be outstanding communicators and are able to work as part of a team in high pressure situations.

Typical International Baccalaureate requirements: 30 points.

Typical A-levels requirements: ABB.

Typical IELTS requirements: 7.0 overall, with no lower than 6.0 in any one component.

Please note that entry requirements vary for each U.K. university.

Nursing University Rankings

To learn more about the best Nursing courses in the U.K., find details on the top ten ranking Nursing and Midwifery universities in the Guardian University Guide 2020 below:

(1) University of Edinburgh;

(2) University of Liverpool;

(3) University of Glasgow;

(4) Coventry University;

(5) University of Portsmouth;

(6) Keele University;

(7) Swansea University;

(8) University of Manchester;

(9) University of Northumbria;

(10) University of Birmingham.

2. Project 2

Viewpoint: When one applies for a university overseas, should he / she place Overall Ranking over Subject Ranking, or should it be the other way round? Respond with your own opinion.

Section E

Self-assessment【进阶评估 自我超越】

1. Cooperative Learning Assessment

Please check your contribution to the group after the project is done.

	Superior (5)	Above Average (4)	Average (3)	Below Average (2)	Weak (1)
Understood what was required for the project					
Participated in the group discussion					
Helped the group to function well as a team					
Contributed useful ideas					

	Superior (5)	Above Average (4)	Average (3)	Below Average (2)	Weak (1)
How much work was done					
Quality of completed work					
What could you improve upon next time?					
Your group members' comments					
Your group leader's comments					

2. Assessment of Individual Study

Instructions:

(1) Read each statement in the table below and place a check mark in the column that best describes how well you can complete that task.

(2) Review your responses for each task. If you have checked five or more in the "Somewhat" and / or "No" columns, you may need to consider making greater efforts after class.

I can	Yes	Somewhat	No
Understand the main idea of the text			
Identify the major points, important facts and details, and vocabulary in the text			
Make inferences about what is implied in the text			
Recognize the organization and purpose of the text			
Remember the new words and expressions			
Speak on the topic effectively			
Employ search strategy to gain information to address the project			
Refer to appropriate resources to deal with the project			

3. Personal Development

Instruction:

Completing this section will help you make informed practicing decisions. Please identify your strengths and the areas that you need to develop or strengthen and record them below.

STRENGTHS: I am confident that I can...
(1)
(2)
(3)

AREAS FOR IMPROVEMENT: I would like to improve my ability to...
(1)
(2)
(3)

Unit 3　Health Professionals in an International Context
"医"者无疆

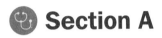

Section A

Warm-up Activity【职业选择　专业态度】

Before a healthcare professional starts planning his / her international career, it is necessary that he / she rethink about the choice. Let's take nursing for example. Why nursing? And what does it mean to be a Nurse? In this video Stanford Health Care nurses talk about why they became a nurse, what being a nurse means to them, what type of person becomes a nurse, and why they love their job. Watch the video "What It Means to Be a Nurse"（Video 6-8）and respond with your own ideas.

Video 6-8

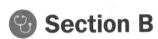

Section B

I　Review and Critical Thinking【创新观点　批判思维】

Working with different patients in different cultures will expose a nurse to more types of medical treatment and procedures, and help her/him communicate better with all kinds of patients. Some nurses choose to go abroad-traveling the world and taking care of patients in other countries, or aiding underserved nations where learned and experienced professional nurses are in high demand. Like all nurses, these men and women are passionate in their desire to help others and are champions of the nursing profession.

Nursing as a Global Profession

Experts agree that today's nurses are essential to the international health perspective. Today's nurse—whether in Baltimore, Beirut or Bangkok-is a global nurse.

A global nurse is culturally sensitive, collaborative（协作的）, and knows that conditions like heart disease, cancer, obesity（肥胖）, diabetes（糖尿病）, and infections（感染）have no borders. A global nurse understands that technology has created a smaller world, with people in instant contact and eager to share information. A global nurse knows that what happens in one part of the world affects the others, including the U.S.

Let's start with the basics: What is global health? According to the Consortium（联盟）of Universities for Global Health, the term indicates an area of study, research, and practice that places a priority on improving health and achieving equity in health for all people worldwide. Anne Marie Rafferty's definition—"Global health is concerned with systems, the interdependence (相互依存) between them and how they impact on the experience of healthcare at local, national and international levels"—adds an interactive infrastructure (基础结构) to the definition and is further expanded on by Martha Hill: "It's also about long-term relationships that are mutually beneficial and addressing (应对) issues that span (跨越) borders."

Thomas Quinn notes that it "...incorporates multiple disciplines, interdisciplinary approaches to solving the health problems of the world... It's not limited to one field. It belongs to all fields of expertise (专长，专技), directly or indirectly related to healthcare and health well-being for all people.

The health of everyone on the globe is obviously interconnected, but why should nurses, in particular, care about global health? "Nursing is integral to (对……不可或缺) the definition of global health," says Quinn. "Nurses can play a more important role than just providing the care. They can help shape policy about how care should be given and develop best-case scenarios (设想；情景) for improvement in life and building the health capacity of a country." But being a global nurse, he says, doesn't necessarily mean practicing nursing "beyond the borders of the U.S." It can also mean being a nurse in your own community. "It's still practicing health equity and that's the common denominator (共性) of the issues," he says.

Whether working at home or abroad, having a global perspective—and experience—can offer nurses opportunities to grow and to serve, says Huda Abu-Saad Huijer: "International experience for nurses presents a powerful and rewarding option in addressing leadership development challenges, both global and domestic."

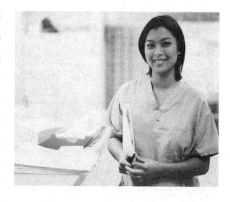

So taking part in global initiatives (全球行动) benefits nurses too? Absolutely, says Hill: "It provides growth opportunities in terms of how we see ourselves, the world, and how we interact." Participating globally provides "stunning and exciting" opportunities to "learn, partner, innovate, collaborate, and build capacity," she says. Practicing abroad or working with international partners can "enhance one's career, and you thrive with (通过……茁壮成长) the intellectual and professional relationships and opportunities."

Sabina De Geest calls this "bringing scientific oxygen to the system." She believes that "by experiencing different systems, you will have a better appreciation of your own system." Experiencing these different systems, adds Mary Woolley, is an ongoing educational opportunity: "We can learn from experiences in a nation other than the U.S. and bring it back home. The learning can go the other direction as well. It needs to be constantly informing, so problem solving can take place."

That kind of international collaboration sounds really rewarding (有回报的). What can nurses do to help improve global health? "The possibilities are endless for nurses in global health. They range from providing an educational role to doing research in a focused way," says Gail Cassell, alluding to (提及) a wide variety of opportunities for nurses to make a difference. The common thread among them, she says, is that "nurses bring a patient-centered focus to the global health team."

Rafferty also spoke to the value that a nurse's perspective offers: "Global nurses practice in a way that is consistent with the values, mindsets (理念), and behaviors associated with global citizenship and play a role in leading change, promoting what I'd call cosmopolitan (世界性的) values in a sustainable (可持续的) way."

Nursing has an "untapped potential (未开发的潜能)," says John Daly. In his view, nurses are able to "develop and implement models of care which will contribute to the renewal (革新) and strategic development of sustainable, quality primary care. Well-educated nurses are well positioned to contribute to health system reforms and healthcare capacity development."

Ⅱ Notes【说文解字　名词注释】

1. Vocabulary Table

Vocabulary 6-3

Words & Expressions	Part of Speech	Meaning in Text
collaborative	*adj.*	协作的
obesity	*n.*	肥胖
diabetes	*n.*	糖尿病
infection	*n.*	感染;传染
Consortium	*n.*	联盟;联合体
interdependence	*n.*	相互依存
infrastructure	*n.*	基础结构;基础设施
address	*vt.*	处理;对付
span	*vt.*	跨越
expertise	*n.*	专业知识;专长;专技
be integral to	*phr.*	对……不可或缺
scenario	*n.*	设想;情景
common denominator	*phr.*	共性
global initiative	*phr.*	全球行动(倡议)
thrive with	*phr.*	借由……而茁壮成长
rewarding	*adj.*	有回报的
alluding to	*phr.*	提及
mindset	*n.*	心态,理念
cosmopolitan	*adj.*	世界性的
sustainable	*adj.*	可持续的
untapped potential	*phr.*	未开发的潜能
renewal	*n.*	革新

2. Useful Knowledge

(1) The Consortium of Universities for Global Health (CUGH), established in 2008, is a membership-based nonprofit organization focusing on global health. Its members are primarily institutions, although individuals can also become members. CUGH members currently include over 145 academic institutions and other organizations.

(2) Although nursing practice varies both through its various specialties and countries, these nursing organizations offer the following definitions:

Nursing encompasses autonomous and collaborative care of individuals of all ages, families, groups and communities, sick or well, and in all settings. Nursing includes the promotion of health, prevention of illness, and the care of ill, disabled and dying people. Advocacy, promotion of a safe environment, research, participation in shaping health policy and in patient and health systems management, and education are also key nursing roles.

— International Council of Nurses

Nursing is the protection, promotion, and optimization of health and abilities; prevention of illness and injury; alleviation of suffering through the diagnosis and treatment of human responses; and advocacy in health care for individuals, families, communities, and populations.

— American Nurses Association

The unique function of the nurse is to assist the individual, sick or well, in the performance of those activities contributing to health or its recovery (or to peaceful death) that he would perform unaided if he had the necessary strength, will or knowledge.

— Virginia Avenel Henderson

(3) The role of patient education in nursing is indispensable. As Benjamin Franklin said, "Tell me and I forget. Teach me and I remember. Involve me and I learn." One of the most important roles a nurse has is in educating patients and their families. The American Nurses Association and the International Council of Nurses consider patient education to be a professional responsibility. Incorporating patient teaching into the plan of care can improve a nurse's teaching effectiveness and increase the likelihood of optimal patient outcomes.

Healthcare's focus has moved from a disease-centered model to one that is patient-centered. Patients are viewed as experts with special knowledge about their own health and preferences for treatments, health states, and outcomes. The primary role of healthcare providers is to assist patients in understanding the significance of health risks and the importance of change. They serve as patient educators and supporters to better aid patient progress in adopting the needed healthy behaviors.

Interdisciplinary involvement by the total healthcare team is central to effective patient care. Ineffective communication among disciplines, patients and family members can create barriers and has even been associated with medication-related adverse events. Nurses have unlimited opportunities to assist patients in managing their health. They

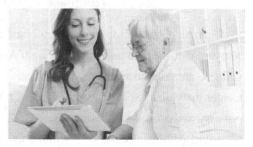

spend more time with patients than any other discipline.

These interactions provide opportunities to develop trust, assess learning needs, and provide continuity throughout the learning process. Members of interdisciplinary teams view nurses as their eyes and ears. They can provide feedback about patient participation, share information that can help team members plan and adjust goals, and reinforce teaching that has been provided.

(4) Primary care is the day-to-day healthcare given by a health care provider. Typically this provider acts as the first contact and principal point of continuing care for patients within a healthcare system, and coordinates other specialist care that the patient may need. Patients commonly receive primary care from professionals such as a primary care physician (general practitioner or family physician), a nurse practitioner (adult-gerontology nurse practitioner, family nurse practitioner, or pediatric nurse practitioner), or a physician assistant. In some localities, such a professional may be a registered nurse, a pharmacist, a clinical officer (as in parts of Africa), or a Ayurvedic or other traditional medicine professional (as in parts of Asia). Depending on the nature of the health condition, patients may then be referred for secondary or tertiary care.

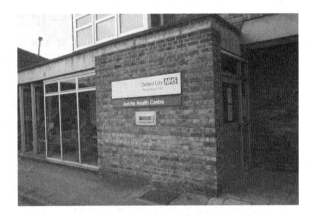

Primary care may be provided in community health centres.

🩺 Section C

Ⅰ Enhanced Learning【深度学习　瓶颈突破】

Language Top Obstacle to Foreign Nurses

Language is the top concern among Chinese nurses who want to work overseas, says Sun Meiyan, who worked as a nurse in Saudi Arabia for seven years. The 33-year-old is now training Chinese nurses who want to work in Saudi Arabia at the Shandong International Nurse Training Center in Weihai, Shandong province. "English medical terms can be very challenging and it's not easy to master them," Sun says.

Sun, who majored in foreign nursing care, went through a three-month language course at the Weihai training center before working at the Almana General Hospital in Al-Hofuf, the first overseas hospital she worked at. But she still faced many difficulties in communicating with patients during the first three months. "The first thing we did after getting off work was to summarize and memorize new words we learned that day," Sun says. "Usually, it will take a Chinese nurse at least six months to communicate well with the patients who will not slow down their speech just because you are a foreign nurse. If you speak good English, you will be more competitive than other applicants in the job interviews."

When interviewers from Saudi German Hospital came to Weihai to hire nurses, they chose Sun without hesitation after knowing that she had worked in Almana General Hospital for five years. Sun instructs her students to focus on language. Besides English, nurses who want to work in Saudi Arabia need to learn some Arabic. "We give them 12-hour training sessions on simple Arabic before they leave for Saudi Arabia, as most elderly people in Saudi Arabia speak only Arabic," Sun says.

She also shares knowledge on local laws and culture with her students. "Thanks to the seven -year experience in Saudi Arabia, I understand the country's laws, culture and lifestyle very well," Sun says. Sun always tells each of her students to pay attention to their image and protect patients' privacy. "The uniform should be washed and ironed every day," she says. "In Saudi Arabia, a nurse's image is as important as her professional skills."

(*Source: China Daily Europe*, 08 Aug. 2014)

II Extensive Learning【拓展学习　媒体动态】

Editor's Note: Over the course of time, I have come to see how easy it is to believe that what we believe and what we do medically in the United States must generally be the way medicine is viewed and practiced in most countries.

We hope, therefore, that the readers will be interested every so often to hear physicians around the world describe their medical practices, so that we all may better understand the wide range of what physicians do.

This issue's contribution is from Einer Helander, MD, PhD, a distinguished Swedish physician, trained as a cardiologist and biochemist, who has spent much of his professional life as Chief Physician for the World Health Organization, visiting countries most of us would not consider going to, and spending his time there among the destitute and the disabled.

Read more from
Einar Helander, 2006.

Read more 6-9

Member Profile

Health Volunteers Overseas (HVO) is a private non-profit organization based in Washington D.C. committed to improving healthcare in developing countries through training and education. By emphasizing teaching, HVO aims to create an indigenous group of trained health workers who can teach others. This builds an ongoing capability that will benefit the population long after the volunteer has departed. It has projects in Africa, Asia, Latin America, Eastern Europe, and the Caribbean. Currently, HVO supports over 60 projects in more than 25 countries. Each project is different depending on the technological capacity of the country.

Main Activities

HVO is a teaching and training organization. Volunteers lecture, conduct ward rounds and demonstrate various techniques in classrooms, clinics, and operating rooms. They may be involved in teacher training, curriculum development, and mentoring of students. These providers can be in the following specialties: anesthesia, dermatology, internal medicine, oral and maxillofacial surgery, orthopaedics, pediatrics, hand surgeons. These highly skilled and experienced volunteers come from both private practice and university settings, with a significant number of retirees as well.

Read more from
WHO, 2019

Read more 6-10

China is planning to open more Confucius Institutes to teach traditional Chinese medicine (TCM) overseas in order to promote this age-old medical science, deemed the essence of Chinese culture, said Vice Minister of Health Wang Guoqiang.

Wang, who is also director of the State Administration of TCM, said Monday: "We are working closely with the Ministry of Education and the Confucius Institute headquarters to open more TCM Confucius Institutes and add TCM courses to the syllabus of existing Confucius Institutes,"

"TCM is very well received abroad, regardless of nationality or ideology," Wang said. However, he added, China lacks talented practitioners who have both a good command of TCM and speak a foreign language.

The Confucius Institutes, named after the ancient Chinese philosopher, are non-profit public institutions for promoting Chinese language and culture in foreign countries.

Read more from
China Daily, 2019

Read more 6-11

Program taps Chinese nurses to plug staffing shortages in the West.

A young Chinese nurse boarded a flight on Aug 3 to start living her dream. The 25-year-old, who specializes in foreign nursing care, flew with seven other Chinese nurses to Stuttgart, Germany, to work at a residential care center for at least three years.

Xie Yanxi is one of the nurses benefiting from a program signed by China and Germany at the end of 2012. The program aimed to recruit 150 Chinese nurses in the following three years to work in Germany.

Faced with an aging society and a shortage of nurses, countries including Australia, Japan, Canada, Singapore and New Zealand have turned to Chinese healthcare professionals to help plug the gap.

The program marked the first time Germany recruited Chinese nurses, providing precious opportunities and possibly opening more of these for Chinese healthcare professionals who want to work in Europe.

Read more from
China Daily, 2014

Read more 6–12

Many give up their careers in China because of low pay and few benefits.

Nurse Song Yan would have sought a job in another country if not for her family and child.

"I work at least nine hours a day and overtime from time to time, and get meager pay," said the veteran nurse who has practiced the profession for at least 20 years.

"The working environment here is noisy, crowded and sometimes even chaotic," said Song, a senior nurse at the chest surgery department of Xuanwu Hospital Capital Medical University in Beijing.

For young nurses, the work is even tougher. "They usually have to work extra to gain patients' trust," she noted.

Read more from
China Daily, 2013

Read more 6–13

Medical workers are broadening their horizons, as Yang Wanli reports in Hamburg and Tang Yue in Beijing.

Song Xi, a 24-year-old nurse, is planning her trip to Germany, but the preparations have been far from easy.

She has only been abroad once before, to Vietnam, and this time her journey will not be a short sightseeing trip, but a working visit for three to five years.

When it comes to hiring nurses, turning to Chinese recruits is nothing new.

As many countries face the problem of an aging society and difficulties in hiring nurses—due to work stress and low wages—employing Chinese workers has become popular in some Asian countries including Singapore, Japan and South Korea.

Read more from
China Daily, 2013

Read more 6-14

Video Resources for Extensive Learning

(1) A day in the life of an ICU nurse. (Video 6-9)
(2) Secret life of male nurses. (Video 6-10)

Video 6-9

Video 6-10

Section D

Projects in Practice【实践探索 行动项目】

1. Project 1

Interview: When we asked Julie A. Green, RN, to describe a typical day in her life as a medical-surgical (med-surg) nurse, she couldn't help but laugh. Our interview with her revealed that each day for a med-surg nurse is anything but typical. Read on to get a glimpse into Green's experience in the fast-paced, team-based, patient-oriented world of med-surg nursing. (Script: A Day in the Life of One Medical-Surgical Nurse)

Now work with your group members for a 5-min presentation based upon the passage "A Day in the Life of One Medical-Surgical Nurse", and provide your answers to "What are must-have skills for medical professionals in a globalized context".

Resource 6-1

2. Project 2

Viewpoint: Today there are many medical professionals specializing in profitable activities such as plastic surgery and private health care for privileged patients. Should doctors and nurses, however, be concentrating more on the general public's health, regardless of how rich patients may be? What is your opinion?

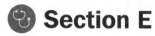 Section E

Self-assessment【进阶评估　自我超越】

1. Cooperative Learning Assessment

Please check your contribution to the group after the project is done.

	Superior (5)	Above Average (4)	Average (3)	Below Average (2)	Weak (1)
Understood what was required for the project					
Participated in the group discussion					
Helped the group to function well as a team					
Contributed useful ideas					
How much work was done					
Quality of completed work					
What could you improve upon next time?					
Your group members' comments					
Your group leader's comments					

2. Assessment of Individual Study

Instructions:

(1) Read each statement in the table below and place a check mark in the column that best describes how well you can complete that task.

(2) Review your responses for each task. If you have checked five or more in the "Somewhat" and / or "No" columns, you may need to consider making greater efforts after class.

I can	Yes	Somewhat	No
Understand the main idea of the text			
Identify the major points, important facts and details, and vocabulary in the text			
Make inferences about what is implied in the text			
Recognize the organization and purpose of the text			
Remember the new words and expressions			
Speak on the topic effectively			
Employ search strategy to gain information to address the project			
Refer to appropriate resources to deal with the project			

3. Personal Development

Instruction:

Completing this section will help you make informed practicing decisions. Please identify your strengths and the areas that you need to develop or strengthen and record them below.

STRENGTHS:
I am confident that I can...

(1)

(2)

(3)

AREAS FOR IMPROVEMENT:
I would like to improve my ability to...

(1)

(2)

(3)

图书在版编目（CIP）数据

医疗通识英语 / 崔红, 洪洋主编. — 杭州：浙江大学出版社，2020.11（2022.11重印）

ISBN 978-7-308-20642-6

Ⅰ.①医… Ⅱ.①崔… ②洪… Ⅲ.①医学－英语 Ⅳ.①R

中国版本图书馆CIP数据核字(2020)第189907号

医疗通识英语

主编　崔　红　洪　洋

责任编辑　李　晨

责任校对　陈丽勋

封面设计　春天书装

出版发行　浙江大学出版社

　　　　　（杭州市天目山路148号　邮政编码310007）

　　　　　（网址：http://www.zjupress.com）

排　　版　杭州兴邦电子印务有限公司

印　　刷　浙江省邮电印刷股份有限公司

开　　本　787mm×1092mm　1/16

印　　张　15

字　　数　500千

版 印 次　2020年11月第1版　2022年11月第3次印刷

书　　号　ISBN 978-7-308-20642-6

定　　价　48.00元

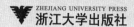

互联网+教育+出版

立方书

教育信息化趋势下，课堂教学的创新催生教材的创新，互联网+教育的融合创新，教材呈现全新的表现形式——教材即课堂。

 轻松备课　 分享资源　 发送通知　 作业评测　 互动讨论

"一本书"带来"一个课堂"　教学改革从"扫一扫"开始

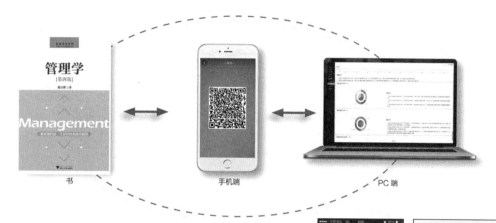

书　　　　　　　　手机端　　　　　　　　PC端

打造中国大学课堂新模式

【创新的教学体验】

开课教师可免费申请"立方书"开课，利用本书配套的资源及自己上传的资源进行教学。

【方便的班级管理】

教师可以轻松创建、管理自己的课堂，后台控制简便，可视化操作，一体化管理。

【完善的教学功能】

课程模块、资源内容随心排列，备课、开课，管理学生、发送通知、分享资源、布置和批改作业、组织讨论答疑、开展教学互动。

扫一扫　下载APP

教师开课流程

➡ 在APP内扫描封面二维码，申请资源

➡ 开通教师权限，登录网站

➡ 创建课堂，生成课堂二维码

➡ 学生扫码加入课堂，轻松上课

网站地址：www.lifangshu.com

技术支持：lifangshu2015@126.com；电话：0571-88273329